# An Orthopaedics Guide for Today's GP

# An Orthopaedics Guide for Today's GP

Edited by

**Maneesh Bhatia**
University Hospitals of Leicester
Leicester, UK

**Tim Jennings**
Syston Health Centre
Leicester, UK

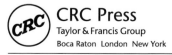

CRC Press
Taylor & Francis Group
Boca Raton London New York

CRC Press is an imprint of the
Taylor & Francis Group, an **informa** business

CRC Press
Taylor & Francis Group
6000 Broken Sound Parkway NW, Suite 300
Boca Raton, FL 33487-2742

Printed on acid-free paper

International Standard Book Number-13: 978-1-78523-126-1 (Paperback)

### Library of Congress Cataloging-in-Publication Data

Names: Bhatia, Maneesh, editor. | Jennings, Tim (Timothy Robin), 1959- editor.
Title: An orthopaedics guide for today's GP / [edited by] Maneesh Bhatia and Tim Jennings.
Description: Boca Raton : CRC Press, [2017] | Includes bibliographical references.
Identifiers: LCCN 2017001552 (print) | LCCN 2017003785 (ebook) | ISBN 9781785231261 (pbk. : alk. paper) | ISBN 9781138048928 (hardback : alk. paper) | ISBN 9781315384030 (Master eBook)
Subjects: | MESH: Musculoskeletal Diseases—diagnosis | Musculoskeletal Diseases—therapy | General Practice—methods
Classification: LCC RC925.5 (print) | LCC RC925.5 (ebook) | NLM WE 140 | DDC 616.7—dc23
LC record available at https://lccn.loc.gov/2017001552

**Visit the Taylor & Francis Web site at**
http://www.taylorandfrancis.com

**and the CRC Press Web site at**
http://www.crcpress.com

I would like to dedicate this book to Juhi, Yash, Sulaxni and our parents.

**Maneesh Bhatia**

# Contents

# Foreword

I am delighted to endorse this short practical guide to orthopaedic conditions in general practice on behalf of the Royal College of General Practitioners. Many of our patients will experience musculoskeletal and orthopaedic problems during the course of their lives, and caring for such patients makes a substantial contribution to our daily workload. This eminently sensible and practical guide helps us to care for our patients with orthopaedic problems and provides an excellent resource for GPs in training and newly qualified GPs as well as the established practitioner. It is the product of a close working relationship between a GP and a consultant orthopaedic surgeon based on a well-established educational programme for GPs delivered as part of their continuing professional development. It is therefore highly topical and relevant to our daily practice. A wide range of healthcare professionals have contributed chapters ranging from consultant orthopaedic surgeons through rheumatologists, physiotherapists and general practitioners. The clinical areas covered are comprehensive and include paediatric orthopaedic issues, hip, knee, foot and ankle disorders as well as bone and soft tissue tumours. I have no doubt that this book will have an important place on the GP's desk for many years to come, and the authors are to be congratulated on producing this high quality and timely book.

**Nigel Mathers MD, PhD, FRCGP**
Honorary Secretary RCGP
Professor of Primary Medical Care
University of Sheffield

# Preface: Maneesh Bhatia

Being married to a general practitioner (GP), I have a fair understanding about the high pressure and demanding role which today's GPs are expected to cope with. Musculoskeletal conditions constitute a big chunk of their day-to-day practice. Although there are a number of online resources with vast amount of theory, these are not catered to help a GP running a busy clinic who needs advice regarding management of a patient in front of him/her.

I have a special interest in GP education and have been running musculoskeletal examination and joint injection courses for last 5–6 years. Talking to a number of GP colleagues and friends, it became quite obvious that there is a need for a concise, practical book that GPs can use as a convenient reference for all musculoskeletal problems. This has inspired me to write a book which fulfils this need. A group of musculoskeletal consultants who are masters in their sub-speciality along with primary care GPs actively involved in GP education have contributed to this project. I hope this book will serve as a valuable tool to those working in or planning to join primary care, and also to medical students as an introduction to orthopaedic practice.

# Preface: Tim Jennings

I asked Maneesh Bhatia to run a teaching session for my GP registrars on our Half Day Release Programme on Foot and Ankle Orthopaedic Problems. This had been highlighted as a learning need, and an interactive session was highly valued. After the session he told me about his idea for this book, and I was keen to be involved.

GPs are under increasing pressure to reduce unnecessary referrals, A&E attendances and admissions. Musculoskeletal (MSK) problems are a daily presentation to the GP – from children, through the sporting adult into the degenerative problems of the elderly. Up-to-date, reliable, easy-to-access information is key for us. As a busy GP, I find Internet resources can be too lay orientated and simplistic, or difficult to assess for bias and reliability in a global healthcare market. I see this book as a must-have resource just like the BNF I still reach for on a daily basis.

Orthopaedic problems regularly feature as cases in the Clinical Skills Assessment exam for membership of the Royal College of General Practitioners (MRCGP). This book will provide history and examination skills with up-to-date management advice for those problems.

# Editors

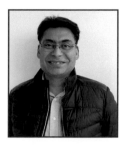

**Maneesh Bhatia** is a consultant orthopaedic, foot and ankle surgeon at the University Hospitals of Leicester, Leicester, United Kingdom. Following training in South East Thames, London, he did a one-year fellowship in foot and ankle surgery at Cambridge. He was awarded the European Travelling Foot & Ankle Fellowship to the USA in 2009. He is on the editorial board of a couple of scientific journals and an examiner for the Royal College of Surgeons. He has acted in the role of specialist advisor to the National Institute for Health and Care Excellence (NICE) regarding treatment of Achilles tendon ruptures. He is a member of the advisory panel of the National Institute for Health Research (NIHR). He has a keen interest in GP teaching and runs joint injection and musculoskeletal core examination skills courses.

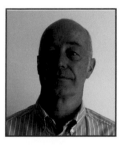

**Tim Jennings** qualified from Guy's Hospital, London, in 1981. He did his general practice Vocational Training Scheme (VTS) training in Leicester from 1982 to 1985. He joined Syston Health Centre, Leicester, as a GP partner in 1985 and continues to work there. He became a GP trainer in 1990. He was appointed the programme director of Health Education East Midlands (HEEM) in 1990 and is still thriving in this role today. He is a school medical officer.

# Contributors

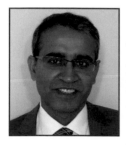

**Sanjeev Anand** is a consultant orthopaedic surgeon with a special interest in knees, sports injuries and hip arthroscopy at Leeds Teaching Hospitals NHS Trust, Leeds, United Kingdom. He is an honorary senior lecturer, Leeds University, Middlesbrough, United Kingdom. He is the editor-in-chief of the *Journal of Arthroscopy and Joint Surgery*. He is an executive member-at-large of the British Association for Surgery of the Knee (BASK).

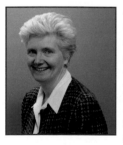

**Alison Armstrong** was appointed a consultant orthopaedic and trauma surgeon in 1997 at the University Hospitals of Leicester NHS Trust, Leicester, United Kingdom, with an interest in shoulder and elbow surgery. She has held posts at national level for the British Orthopaedic Directors Society (Chairman), Professional Practice Committee of BOA and Education Committee of BESS. Currently she is an FRCS Orth Examiner and Divisional Research Lead.

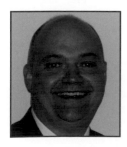

**Robert U Ashford** is a consultant orthopaedic and musculoskeletal tumour surgeon at Leicester Orthopaedics and the East Midlands Sarcoma Service. His specialist interest is the surgical management of metastatic malignancy and palliative orthopaedic surgery. His research interests include the genetic causes of soft-tissue sarcoma, outcomes after treatment of soft-tissue sarcoma, desmoid fibromatosis and the management of skeletal metastases.

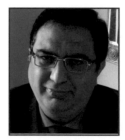

**Sunil Bajaj** is a consultant orthopaedic surgeon with special interest in paediatric orthopaedics. He works at Queen Elizabeth Hospital Woolwich, Queen Mary's Hospital Sidcup, University Hospital Lewisham. Bajaj has written chapters for many books including *Mercer's Textbook of Orthopaedics*.

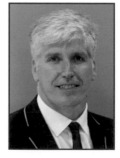

**Kevin Boyd** is a consultant orthopaedic and sports injuries surgeon at the University Hospitals of Leicester NHS Trust, Leicester, United Kingdom. He was trained in Newcastle-upon-Tyne, Nottingham and Brisbane, Australia, and is a Fellow of the Royal College of Surgeons of England and of the Faculty of Sport & Exercise Medicine of the United Kingdom. He has active roles in research, teaching and examining, both locally and internationally.

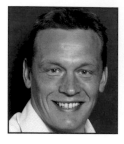

**Jason Braybrooke** is a consultant orthopaedic spine surgeon in Leicester. He went to Leicester Medical School as an undergraduate and remained in Leicester for his Higher Surgical Training. He completed a fellowship at the Sunnybrook and Women's in Toronto, Canada and has been a Consultant in Leicester since 2008.

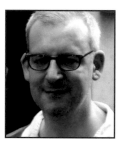

**Philip N Green** has been a full-time GP and partner at Syston Health Centre, Leicestershire, Leicester, United Kingdom, for the last 15 years, having graduated from the Leicester University School of Medicine in 1996 and thereafter, the Leicester GP Training Scheme in 2001. Phil is proud to be a member of the Teenage Cancer Trust and has spent a number of years offering counselling to young cancer sufferers, particularly those with bone cancers.

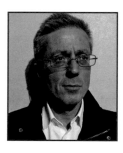

**Tim Green** has just retired after working for 21 years as a consultant orthopaedic knee surgeon. He worked as a roofer before studying medicine in Birmingham. He has a wealth of experience and worked in Birmingham, Stoke on Trent, Gloucester and Bristol before his appointment as a consultant at Leicester in 1995.

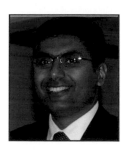

**Vikas Khanduja** is a consultant orthopaedic surgeon at Addenbrookes Cambridge University Hospital NHS Trust. He specializes in hip and knee surgery and has a particular interest in hip arthroscopy. He is the Director of the MCh (Orth) Programme at the Anglia Ruskin University, East Anglia, United Kingdom. He is an associate editor of the *Bone and Joint Journal* and a reviewer for many scientific orthopaedic journals.

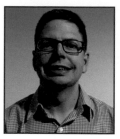

**Ralph Leighton** is a consultant anaesthetist at the University Hospitals of Leicester NHS Trust, Leicester, United Kingdom. He graduated in London and subsequently was trained in the East Midlands. His special interests include pre-operative assessment, medical education and obstetric anaesthesia.

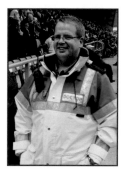

**Stephen Le Maistre** was trained at Charing Cross and Westminster Medical School, graduating in 1998. He joined the GP vocational training scheme in Northampton in 2000. Stephen is a partner at Langham Place Surgery, and also the crowd doctor for Northampton Town FC.

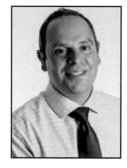

**Nicolas Nicolaou** is a consultant paediatric orthopaedic surgeon at Sheffield Children's Hospital, Sheffield, UK. He qualified from the King's College School of Medicine and Dentistry in 1999 and has a specialist interest in the paediatric knee and paediatric orthopaedic research.

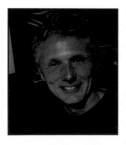

**Tom Rowley** is a GP partner working in Leicester. He has a specialist interest in MSK and sports and exercise medicine, with postgraduate diploma qualifications in these areas. He has worked as a hospital practitioner in orthopaedics, and also ran a primary care MSK service for many years. He is a member and a steering committee representative of the Primary Care Rheumatology Society.

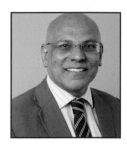

**Ash Samanta** has over 25 years of experience as a consultant rheumatologist at the University Hospitals of Leicester NHS Trust, Leicester, United Kingdom. He has considerable expertise in medical leadership, as well as education and training at undergraduate and postgraduate levels. He is also qualified in law and undertakes medico-legal and medical professional regulatory work at national level. He has published widely in peer-reviewed journals and has co-authored *Rheumatology: A Clinical Handbook, Medical Law* (Palgrave Macmillan) and *Concentrate: Medical Law* (Oxford University Press).

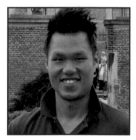

**Matthew Seah** is an NIHR Academic Clinical Fellow and a specialty registrar in orthopaedics and is currently working in Cambridge. His interests in musculoskeletal research include novel therapies for cartilage regeneration/repair in osteoarthritis, as well as the clinical translation of cell therapies for cartilage regeneration.

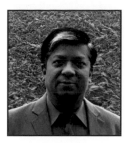

**Bijayendra Singh** is a consultant in trauma and orthopaedics at Medway Foundation NHS Trust. His special interest is the upper limb including hand and wrist disorders. He has an interest in clinical research and has widely published and presented at various national and international meetings.

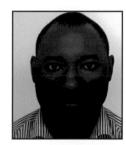

**Kehinde Sunmboye** is a consultant rheumatologist with special interest in vasculitis and connective tissue diseases. He works at the University Hospitals of Leicester, Leicester, United Kingdom.

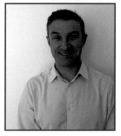

**Richard Wood** is an extended scope musculoskeletal physiotherapist at University Hospitals Leicester, Leicester, United Kingdom, and has more than 20 years of experience with musculoskeletal disorders. He works in a variety of clinical settings including primary care. He has a special interest in lower limb disorders and enjoys teaching.

# 1

# Paediatric orthopaedic disorders

SUNIL BAJAJ and NICOLAS NICOLAOU

# Introduction

It is important to appreciate that not all paediatric deformities, especially of the lower limbs, are pathological. Quite a few of them are physiological and they are referred to as normal variants of lower limb development. These generally spontaneously get better as the child grows. It is important to differentiate normal variants from pathological conditions that present in a similar fashion. The following table provides some differentiating factors:

| Physiological Conditions | Pathological Conditions |
|---|---|
| Usually symmetrical | Rarely symmetrical |
| Flexible deformity – correctable | Rigid deformity |
| Familial (family history positive) | Family history positive or negative |
| Improves with time | Usually worsens with time |
| No active treatment generally necessary | Intervention is almost always needed |

Physiological deformities/normal variants are an important cause of parental concern.

A detailed history and full clinical examination are generally all that is required to differentiate pathological conditions from normal variants.

## What ages do the different normal variants present?

From birth to the first 2 years of life, the following normal variants are present:

1. Packaging deformities
2. Physiological flat foot (pes planus)
3. Physiological bow legs (genu varum)

From 2 years right up to the adolescent age (puberty), the following normal variants are present:

1. Knock knees (genu valgum)
2. In-toeing
3. Out-toeing

## What are packaging defects?

Normal variants which are the result of intrauterine moulding are called packaging deformities. These include:

1. Hyper-extension of the knee
2. Postural talipes/calcaneovalgus foot
3. Out-toeing of infants as a result of external rotator contracture
4. Metatarsus adductus

Below is the brief description of some of the above deformities.

## In-toeing and out-toeing

In-toeing, most commonly known as pigeon toes (Figure 1.1), refers to an inward pointing foot and is more common than out-toeing (foot points outwards) (Figure 1.2). They are an important cause for parental concern and a frequent referral to paediatric orthopaedic clinics. The majority of the cases are physiological (normal variants) and spontaneously resolve with time. It is important to understand how the normal rotational profile of lower limbs changes with the child's age and development.

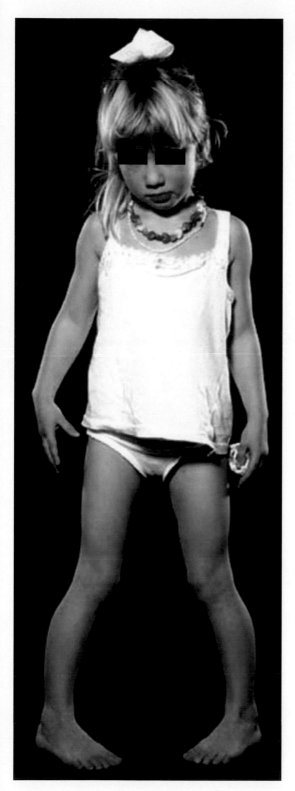

Figure 1.1 Bilateral and symmetrical In-toeing.

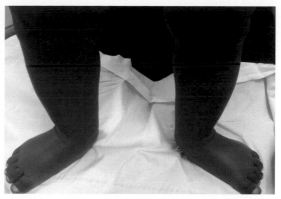

Figure 1.2 Bilateral and symmetrical out-toeing.

## How does the rotational profile of the lower limb change with the age and development of the child?

### Natural History – Rotation

- Limb buds appear in 6-week-old embryo
- Around the eighth week (foetal stage), upper limb rotates 90° externally and lower limb rotates internally
- Subsequent intrauterine moulding results in external hip rotation, internal tibial rotation and variable foot position
- Postnatal period to adolescence – lower limb rotates externally (25° of external rotation in the femur, 15° of external rotation in the tibia)

## What are the causes of in-toeing?

In-toeing is usually physiological (normal variant). Depending on the age of presentation, causes include metatarsus adductus, increased internal tibial torsion and increased or persistent femoral anteversion.

Metatarsus adductus – first 2 years of life
Internal tibial torsion – toddlers to preschoolers
Increased femoral anteversion – school ages children to adolescence

## What is metatarsus adductus?

This is defined as an atypical inward twisting/bending of the foot, also referred to as pigeon toes (Figure 1.3). The lateral border of the foot is curved (Figure 1.4) (assessed by holding a pencil along the lateral border). This is as a result of the intrauterine moulding of the foot (packaging defect). Clinical examination of the feet reveals a symmetrical deformity in both feet. The entire forefoot is adducted at the tarsometatarsal level. The hindfoot is in normal position. The deformity is not rigid and can be passively corrected. It is important to examine the hips in children presenting with metatarsus adductus to rule out developmental dysplasia, which is also a part of the packaging disorders.

## What is the treatment for metatarsus adductus?

Ninety percent of feet correct spontaneously by the age of 1 year and do not require any active treatment. The parents need to be reassured. In moderate-to-severe metatarsus adductus deformity, stretching exercises may help. Referral to a paediatric physiotherapy team can also help. Metatarsus adductus in the older child may require serial casting or splinting. Metatarsus adductus deformity usually resolves by 1 year, though it may persist until 3–4 years of age in some cases.

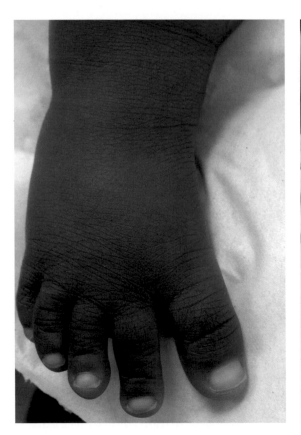

Figure 1.3 Dorsal view of foot with metatarsus adductus.

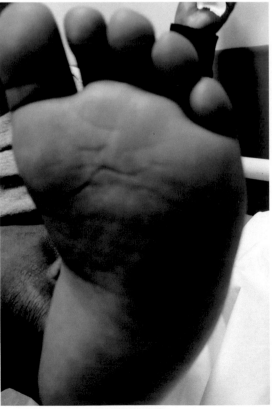

Figure 1.4 Metatarsus adductus with curved lateral border.

## What is congenital metatarsus varus?

This condition is a pathological cause of in-toeing in the first 2 years of life. It should be differentiated from metatarsus adductus. The following are the features which help to differentiate the two:

1. Metatarsus adductus can be corrected by passive manipulation.
2. Absence of the crease in the medial plantar aspect of the foot in metatarsus adductus. A deep medial skin crease is evident on the foot in congenital metatarsus varus (Figure 1.5).

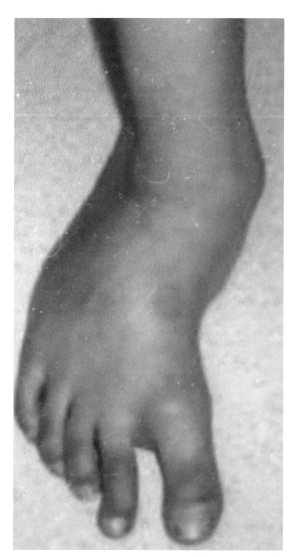

Figure 1.5 Medial crease in Congenital metatarsus varus.

If any of the above features are present, a referral to paediatric orthopaedic surgery should be made, as it may need serial casting or surgery in resistant cases.

## What is internal tibial torsion?

Internal tibial torsion is a common cause of in-toeing in older children (2–3 years of age). Examination would reveal the entire leg is oriented medially from the knee. The deformity is bilaterally symmetrical in both legs.

## How do you assess/measure internal tibial torsion?

Internal tibial torsion may be measured by the thigh-foot angle in the prone position (Figure 1.6).

Normal thigh-foot angle in children ranges from 5° to 20°.

## What is the treatment for internal tibial torsion?

The deformity spontaneously corrects or resolves itself by 3–4 years of age.

Internal tibial torsion if symptomatic (knee pain) may be addressed by derotation osteotomy in the older child (7–8 years of age).

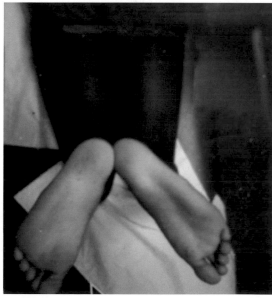

Figure 1.6 Thigh–foot angle measured in the prone position.

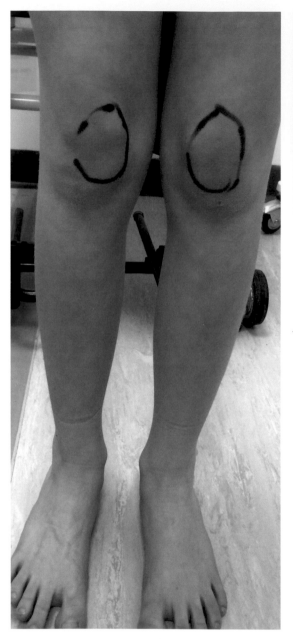

Figure 1.7 Border of the patellae marked showing medial patella squint on the right side.

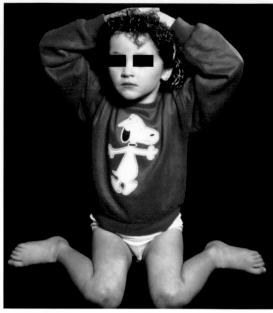

Figure 1.8 Child sitting in 'W' position due to persistent femoral anteversion.

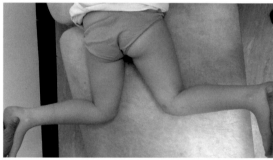

Figure 1.9 Increased internal rotation of the hips seen in excessive femoral anteversion.

the siblings. Clinical examination also reveals in-toeing and a medial patella squint (patella pointing inwards when the child stands or walks) (Figure 1.7).

These children are observed to sit in the typical W position (Figure 1.8).

## What is excessive femoral anteversion?

Excessive femoral anteversion or antetorsion is increased femoral internal rotation. Femoral antetorsion is a common cause of in-toeing in older children between 3 and 5 years of age. It affects girls more than boys and manifests a similar growth pattern for

## How do you measure femoral anteversion?

Femoral anteversion can be measured by assessing internal and external rotation of the child's hip. Internal rotation more than 70° (Figure 1.9) and external rotation of less than 20° suggests femoral anteversion (Figure 1.10).

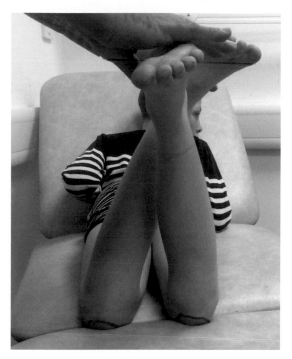

Figure 1.10 Reduced external rotation of the hips seen in excessive femoral anteversion.

## How do you treat the above condition?

Femoral anteversion normally remodels as a child grows. Deformity remodels by 8 years of age. Persistent femoral anteversion, if symptomatic, may warrant a derotation osteotomy of the femur after the age of 8–10 years.

## Is in-toeing always physiological?

No, there are pathological causes for in-toeing. A detailed history and a meticulous clinical examination would help to identify these causes, which include neurological disorders like cerebral palsy, metabolic bone diseases and skeletal dysplasia.

## What is out-toeing?

Out-toeing refers to toes pointing outwards when the child stands or walks, or 'Charlie Chaplin' appearance (Figure 1.11). Out-toeing is much less common than in-toeing. It can occur as a result of packing disorder of the intrauterine moulding resulting in contracture of the external rotator

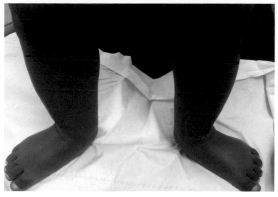

Figure 1.11 Bilateral out-toeing–Charlie Chaplin gait.

muscles of hips. The condition is generally benign and corrects spontaneously, especially when the child starts to walk.

However, the pathological causes of out-toeing include deformities of the foot, such as congenital vertical talus and tarsal coalition. Outward twisting of the leg bone (external tibial torsion) or the hip (femoral retroversion). In the older child (more than 8–10 years of age), it is essential to rule out slipped capital femoral epiphysis (SCFE) which is also associated with femoral retroversion. Pathological causes result in asymmetrical out-toeing and may not spontaneously correct, necessitating surgery if the child is symptomatic.

### POINTS TO REMEMBER

1. In-toeing/out-toeing is a common cause for parenteral concern.
2. It commonly is physiological (normal variant).
3. A detailed history (birth/developmental history and family history) is a must to differentiate it from pathological causes.
4. The majority of cases correct/remodel as the child grows.

## What are bow legs (genu varum) and knock knees (genu valgum)?

Bow legs (Figure 1.12) and knock knees (Figure 1.13) are the common angular deformities of the lower

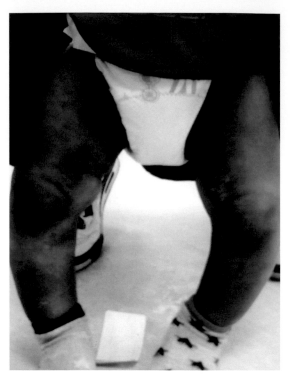

Figure 1.12 Bilateral symmetrical bow legs.

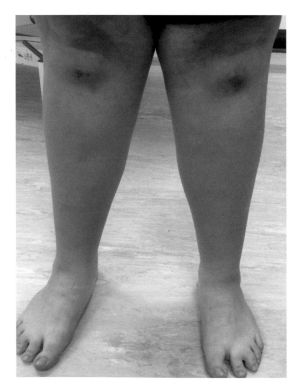

Figure 1.13 Bilateral knock knees (genu valgum).

limbs presenting to general medical practice. It is important to know that the shape of the lower limbs constantly changes as a child grows. Symmetrical bowing of the legs is normal up to the age of 2 years. An increasing valgus attitude of the lower limbs develops from 2 to 4 years of age, giving a knock knee appearance. This reverts to the normal adult alignment at 6–8 years of age. Hence, both bow legs and knock knees are normal processes of a child's development. However, there are pathological causes of above deformities. These include:

1. Trauma
2. Metabolic conditions like rickets
3. Tibia vara – Blount's disease
4. Dysplasia of the skeleton

It is important to differentiate physiological from pathological. This can be done by a good history and focussed clinical examination. The following table shows some of the differences.

| Physiological Bowing | Pathological Bowing |
| --- | --- |
| Deformities bilateral and symmetric | May be unilateral or dissymmetric |
| Deformity tends to correct with time | Progressively worsens with time |
| Physiological genu varum is seen up to 2 years of age (maximum up to 3 years) | Genu varum persisting beyond 3 years is pathological |
| Physiological genu valgum is seen 4–6 years of age | Pathological genu valgum presents in a child under 3 years of age, or if the intermalleolar distance is >8 cm |

## How do you manage bow legs and knock knees?

Physiological deformities are generally asymptomatic and remodel spontaneously as the child grows. Parental reassurance is necessary. Intermalleolar distance (in cases of knock knees) (Figure 1.14) and intercondylar distance (in cases of bow legs) can be measured to monitor progress. Radiographs of the legs are not necessary.

If the deformity becomes symptomatic or is asymmetrical and progressively worsens in the older child, referral to an orthopaedic specialist is necessary. Once established that the deformity is pathological, management includes correction by guided growth technique or osteotomy.

---

### POINTS TO REMEMBER

1. Angular deformities of the knee are part of normal development of the child.
2. History and clinical examination is sufficient to separate physiological from pathological causes. Radiographs are not necessary.

---

## What are the different feet/ toe deformities seen in general practice?

These include:

- Pes planus
- Pes cavus
- Club foot
- Curly toes
- Overlapping toes

## What is pes planus?

Pes planus, also called flat foot, refers to a foot with loss of the medial longitudinal arch (Figure 1.15).

## What are the different types of flat feet?

These can be classified into flexible (corrects on tip-toeing or not weight-bearing) or rigid. The former is usually physiological.

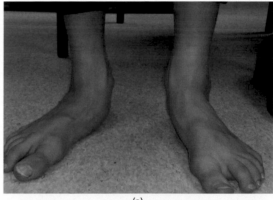

(a)

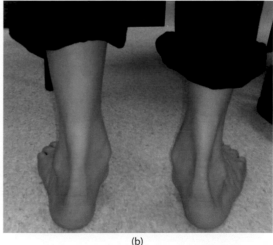

(b)

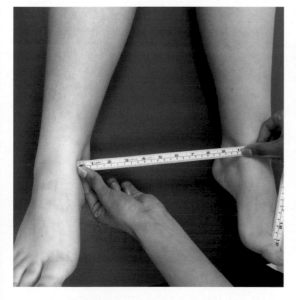

Figure 1.14 Measuring the intermalleolar distance in knock knees.

Figure 1.15 **(a and b)** Bilateral symmetrical pes planus.

## How do we differentiate physiological flat feet from pathological flat feet?

It is important to differentiate physiological flat feet from pathological flat feet. The following table shows some differences.

| Physiological Flat Feet | Pathological Flat Feet |
| --- | --- |
| Flexible | Rigid |
| Always symmetrical | Can be asymmetrical |
| Asymptomatic | Usually painful |
| Usually corrects with time | Usually worsens with time |
| Maintained subtalar/ ankle movements | Subtalar joint stiff |

Flexible flat feet correct (arch appears) on tiptoeing (Figure 1.16).

Flexible flat feet may be associated with a tight gastrocnemius muscle or generalised ligamentous laxity (hypermobile flat foot).

## How do you manage physiological pes planus?

Children with flexible flat feet are usually asymptomatic. They are normally brought by their parents because of concerns about the shape of the feet and the long-term consequences. Most children with physiological or flexible flat feet will develop an arch in the first decade of life, and it is essential to counsel the parents regarding development of arch with the age. However, approximately 20% of individuals will never develop an arch.

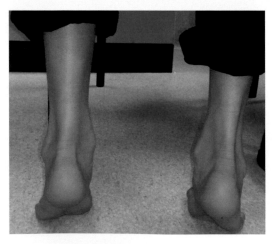

Figure 1.16 Restoration of the foot arch on tiptoeing–flexible flat feet.

The use of orthotics, insoles or modified shoes to treat asymptomatic flexible flat feet has been shown to be ineffective and hence is not recommended.

## What are the causes of rigid flat foot?

Rigid flat foot seen at birth is caused by congenital vertical talus. This has a unique presentation as shown in Figure 1.17a and b.

The heel is in valgus and the foot is dorsiflexed and everted, giving a convex appearance to the sole (rocker-bottom flat foot deformity). The deformity is rigid and not passively correctable. It is usually associated with another musculoskeletal abnormality (syndromic) or may be secondary to neuromuscular problems (e.g. spina bifida, arthrogryposis etc.). Early referral to a paediatric orthopaedic surgeon is necessary.

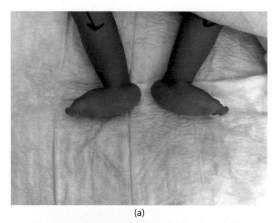

(a)

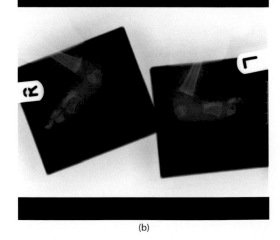

(b)

Figure 1.17 (a) Congenital vertical talus–rocker bottom foot. (b) Lateral radiographs of a rocker bottom foot.

## What is tarsal coalition?

This is a congenital abnormality relating to fusion of tarsal bones and resulting in a rigid flat foot deformity (Figure 1.18). The most common coalition is between the calcaneum and navicular bone and to a lesser extent, between the talus and calcaneum.

## Pathology

The fusion between the tarsal bones may be fibrous, cartilaginous or both. When the subtalar joint movement is restricted by coalition, the distal joints compensate resulting in flattening of the medial arch.

## Clinical presentation

The majority of the tarsal coalitions of patients are asymptomatic. Often the onset of symptoms correlates with the age of ossification of coalition. Generally, navicular coalition presents between the age of 8 and 10 years and talocalcaneal between 10 and 12 years of age. The ankle giving way and pain worsened by activity are the most common symptoms.

Clinical evaluation is essential in rigid flat foot deformity. On inspection, there is a loss of medial longitudinal arch with hindfoot valgus deformity. Forefoot abduction can be appreciated while looking at the feet from the back as 'too many toes sign'. It is essential that patients are asked to stand on their tip-toes and look for correction of the hindfoot valgus deformity. In the absence of correction of deformity on tip-toeing, a diagnosis of rigid flat foot can be made. Subtalar joint movements are restricted or absent.

## Investigation

Osseous tarsal coalition can be diagnosed with simple plain radiographs of the foot (Figure 1.19). Computerised tomography (CT) scans are necessary to determine the size and extent of coalition and also helpful in ruling out additional coalitions. A magnetic resonance imaging (MRI) scan is helpful to visualise the fibrous and cartilaginous coalitions.

## Treatment

In asymptomatic cases, careful monitoring is required. In symptomatic tarsal coalitions, taking a break from high-impact activity for a period of 3–6 weeks can reduce the stress on tarsal bones and relieve pain. Orthotic support such as medial arch support, heel cups and wedges can help to stabilise the foot and relieve the pain. Immobilisation of the foot in a boot or a cast can take the stress off the tarsal bones. Steroid injections can be used in conjunction with other non-surgical treatments to provide temporary symptomatic benefit.

## Surgical treatment

Surgical treatment can be used depending on the time of the diagnosis and the extent of the process. In

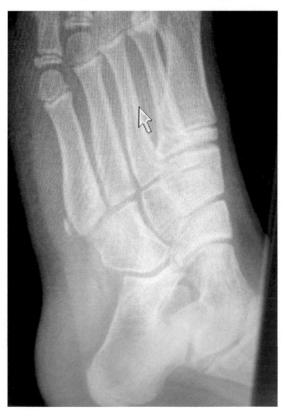

Figure 1.19 Oblique radiographs of the foot demonstrating a calcaneonavicular coalition.

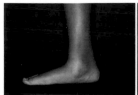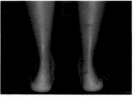

Figure 1.18 Rigid flat foot on the right seen in unilateral tarsal coalition.

symptomatic cases when non-operative management fails to relieve symptoms, surgical resection of the coalition can be performed. The role of a subtalar prosthesis is still questionable; however, in severe advanced cases of coalition, triple arthrodesis may be necessary.

---

**POINTS TO REMEMBER**

1. Flat feet are common in children.
2. The majority are physiological and flexible and asymptomatic.
3. Rigid flat feet are pathological and symptomatic.
4. Insoles/special shoes do not help to correct physiological pes planus.
5. Recurrent ankle sprains with flat feet in an adolescent point to underlying tarsal coalition.

---

## What is pes cavus?

Pes cavus refers to a foot deformity characterised by an elevated medial longitudinal arch. In two-thirds of patients, there may be an associated neurological abnormality such as Charcot Marie tooth, Friedreich's ataxia, cerebral palsy, polio or spinal dysraphism (spinal cord lesions).

## What is the clinical presentation in children with pes cavus?

Children with pes cavus present with pain/ache around the ankle, mid-foot, lateral border of the foot or in the ball of the foot. Pes cavus may be associated with clawing of the toes. In addition, they may also have symptoms of instability in the ankles (ankles giving way) and may have sensory/motor weakness in the limbs if caused by an underlying neurological abnormality.

## How do you manage pes cavus?

Management starts with a detailed history and clinical assessment. Clinical assessment would involve assessment of the foot and also evaluation of the spine to look for spinal dysraphism. In the clinical examination of the foot, one may notice

the obvious deformity of the high medial arch, varus deformity of the heel and also clawing of the toes. A referral to orthopaedic surgery must be made if these features are present. Definitive management depends on symptoms, type of deformity (flexible or rigid) and presence or absence of an underlying neurological problem. Treatment includes physiotherapy, orthotic supports and, if conservative measure fails, surgery.

---

**POINTS TO REMEMBER**

1. Pes cavus is due to a neurological problem unless proved otherwise.
2. Examination of the spine is essential in children with high arch feet.

---

## Osgood–Schlatter disease

This is one of the causes of anterior knee pain in the adolescent age group. It is a traction apophysitis of the tibial tubercle due to stress from the extensor mechanism.

It occurs in adolescent age during a pubertal growth spurt. Affected children are generally males (especially athletes) who complain of pain in the knee (especially localised to the tibial tubercle) commonly following activities like jumping, playing football, coming down stairs etc. Examination reveals swelling and tenderness over the tibial tubercle (Figure 1.20). Symptoms are bilateral in 20%–30% of cases. It is important to examine the hips, as hip pathology like SCFE can present with knee pain in this age group.

Diagnosis is clinical and routine radiographs are not necessary. If symptoms are persistent or there is significant swelling not typical of Osgood–Schlatter disease, x-rays of the knee must be done. Fragmentation of the tibial tubercle physis with soft tissue swelling may be seen on x-ray of the knee (Figure 1.21). Fragmentation should not be mistaken for a fracture.

## What is the management of Osgood–Schlatter disease?

Non-operative management forms the mainstay of the treatment. Education about the fact that the

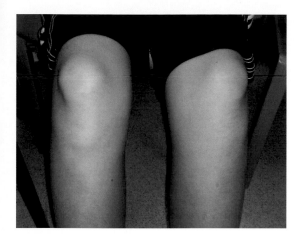

Figure 1.20 Bilateral prominent tibial tubercles in Osgood–Schlatter disease.

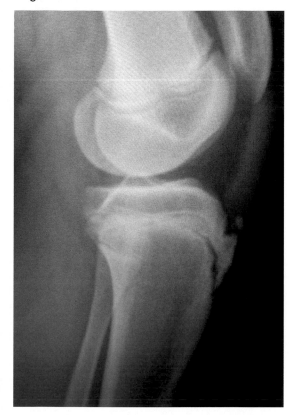

Figure 1.21 Lateral knee radiographs showing fragmentation of tibial tubercle in Osgood–Schlatter disease.

condition will resolve when the physis closes and reassurance of the patient and the parents is essential. During acute exacerbation, rest, ice, analgesia, activity modification (avoiding activities involving traction to tibial tubercle especially jumping/contact sports) and physiotherapy (quadriceps and hamstring stretching) form the mainstay of the treatment. Referral to paediatric physiotherapy is necessary. Orthopaedic referral will be required if physiotherapy fails. In skeletally mature patients, occasional surgery to excise a free ossicle may be necessary.

> ## POINTS TO REMEMBER
>
> 1. Osgood–Schlatter disease is a benign condition common in adolescents.
> 2. Diagnosis is clinical (x-rays are not essential).
> 3. Activity modification and physiotherapy form the mainstay of treatment.
> 4. The condition spontaneously disappears with closure of tibial tubercle physis.

## Is toe walking normal in children?

Toe walking (Figure 1.22) in children is normal up to the age of 2 years. After 2 years, if a child walks on his or her toes, a detailed birth and developmental history to rule out a neuromuscular problem, like cerebral palsy, is essential.

The child needs to be examined to establish the following:

1. Is tip-toe walking constant or occasional?
2. Is it bilateral?
3. Is there a family history of toe walking in other children?
4. Is it associated with tight gastrocnemius or tendo-achilles?
5. Is there evidence of any neurological problem in the lower extremities (examine tone, power, reflexes and sensations in both lower limbs).
6. The spine needs to be examined for any neurocutaneous markers for underlying spinal dysraphism.
7. Is there any evidence of muscular dystrophy (e.g. Duchenne)?

If all the above are ruled out, then it is a case of idiopathic toe walking.

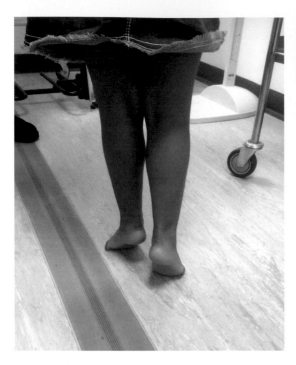

Figure 1.22 Bilateral idiopathic toe walking.

## Management

Management of idiopathic toe walking is difficult. A referral to a paediatric physiotherapist for stretching exercises and gait training is recommended.

A referral to an orthopaedic surgeon would be made by the physiotherapist, if the problem persists. The options of further management include:

1. Serial casting (to sequentially stretch tendo-achilles)
2. Percutaneous tendo-achilles lengthening

It is important to explain to the parents that the child may continue to toe walk in spite of all measures (especially in habitual toe walkers).

## What are curly toes?

Curly toes refer to toe deformities characterised by flexion and medial deviation of the proximal interphalangeal (PIP) joint of the toe. The deformity is bilateral and mainly affects the fourth and fifth toes (Figure 1.23). There is generally a positive family history. Generally, curly toes are asymptomatic but can present with pain and pressure effects on tips of toes, especially when walking.

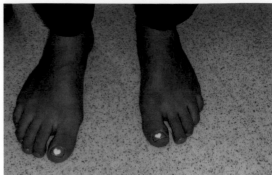

Figure 1.23 Bilateral Curly fourth and fifth toes.

## What causes curly toes?

They are caused by congenital tightness of flexor digitorum longus and brevis (toe flexors).

## How do you manage curly toes?

Education and reassurance of the parents may be all that is required in asymptomatic cases. Twenty-five percent of cases resolve on their own. If symptomatic, referral to a paediatric orthopaedic surgeon is necessary. Surgery involves flexor tenotomy after the age of 3 years.

---

### POINTS TO REMEMBER

1. Toe walking is normal up to age of 2 years.
2. A detailed history and clinical examination to rule out a neuromuscular cause is necessary.
3. Idiopathic (habitual toe walking) is usually associated with tight tendo-achilles.

---

## The paediatric hip

## What is developmental dysplasia of the hip?

This condition represents a spectrum of abnormality ranging from mild acetabular dysplasia to frank dislocation of one or both hips that can present in general practice in varying ages and differing forms. Note that the term 'congenital dislocation of the hip' has been replaced, as in some cases, there is a progression of displacement of the hip with growth, or an improvement that occurs with treatment. Dysplasia untreated has the potential to lead to subluxation of the hip and ultimately dislocation.

## What are the risk factors for this condition to be elicited in the history?

Risk factors for this condition vary in terms of their significance, with some remaining low in both sensitivity and specificity. Breech positioning and family history are considered the most significant. A family history is normally considered an affected first-degree relative treated for the same disorder. Females and first-born children are also risk factors. Developmental dysplasia of the hip (DDH) should also be considered if other intrauterine crowding disorders are present such as torticollis, metatarsus adductus and oligohydramnios. Congenital talipes equinovarus (club foot) is not considered an associated condition.

Primary care physicians will often encounter this disorder during the 24-hour neonatal check or the 6- to 8-week check as advised as part of the Neonatal and Infant Physical Examination (NIPE).

## How do you clinically assess a child with the above risk factors?

Note that the technique of examination differs according to the age of the child. Classical examination of the neonate involves performing the Barlow and Ortolani tests. The most important factor in performance of both of these tests is to have a relaxed child in order to increase identification of pathology. Both of these tests require practice and experience, as this is strongly linked to success in diagnosis.

## Barlow test

This is a provocative test that assesses if a reduced hip is dislocatable. The examination is performed supine on a warm surface; if none is available, then a parent's lap can be used. Both knees are held with the thumb on the inner surface of the thigh. The knees are then gently brought to the midline from an abducted position, with gentle posterior pressure directed towards the hip joint. A positive test occurs when the hip is felt to shift out of the

acetabulum, reducing back into the acetabulum on release of the pressure (Figure 1.24).

## Ortolani test

This assesses if a dislocated hip is reducible, and therefore, is not of use if the hips are located. It can be considered the reverse of the Barlow test, and positioning of the child and placement of the examiners hands is similar. Here, the thumb and index finger stabilise the thigh, while the ring and little finger of the examiner support the greater trochanter. From the midline, both thighs are abducted away from the midline with gentle pressure on the greater trochanter. If the hip is dislocated, a clunk or jump will be felt as the hip reduces into the acetabulum.

Often with the Ortolani and Barlow tests, clicks may be audible but may not be reduction or dislocation. Most clicks that are audible will come from the soft tissue structures around the hip joint, such as the iliotibial band, psoas tendon or the ligamentum teres. Most hips that are positive for the Barlow test will normalise in a few weeks, but as DDH represents a spectrum, ultrasound for positive hips is a good way of excluding dysplasia.

Asymmetrical skin creases often cause concern, particularly amongst health visitors performing hip examination. It is important to note that asymmetry is sensitive for a unilateral dislocation, but not specific. In most cases, this will be a normal variant; 13% of children will have asymmetrical creases on examination. In the absence of risk factors for DDH, or positive clinical signs, it is of doubtful significance in most.

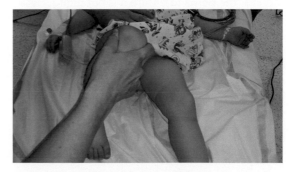

Figure 1.24 Barlow test in an older infant. For screening in a younger child, examination of both hips will take place simultaneously. The leg is brought to the midline with gentle posterior pressure.

In infants older than 3 months, assessment by the Barlow and Ortolani tests is no longer sensitive.

The most reproducible and sensitive clinical sign will be a loss of abduction of the hip. Although this sounds like an easy finding to elicit, often subtle tilting of the pelvis during abduction will give false results. It is therefore essential to ensure a level pelvis when assessing abduction (Figure 1.25).

The Galeazzi sign is a test looking for shortening of the femur that is associated with a hip dislocation. It can be positive with overgrowth conditions such as hemihypertrophy. For this test, the hips are flexed as well as the knees with the feet and knees kept together in the supine position. If the sign is positive, the levels of the knees will be different (Figure 1.26).

Occasionally, children of walking age will present with DDH. In these cases, as the children begin to take their first steps, they may be noted to have a painless limp due to abductor dysfunction. Occasionally, they can present as a unilateral toe walking gait in order to compensate for the

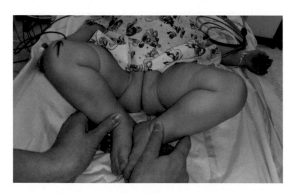

Figure 1.25 Assessment of reduced abduction. Monitor the pelvis to ensure it is not tilting. Here we can see the right hip has a subtle loss of abduction due to dislocation.

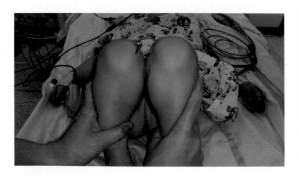

Figure 1.26 Galeazzi test. Note the knees sit at a different height.

shortening of the limb. In these cases, abduction will again be reduced on the affected side, and the Galeazzi sign will be positive. In these older children, bilateral hip dislocations can cause diagnostic difficulty, as the features on each side are often symmetrical. Such children often have a 'waddling gait' in addition to a hyperlordosis of the lumbar spine. Hip abduction will be reduced, showing the importance of this clinical sign in all age groups.

## What is the investigation of choice in a child aged less than 6 months with suspected DDH?

### Ultrasound screening

Selective ultrasound screening for at-risk cases is widely practiced in the United Kingdom, as opposed to the universal screening programme seen in many European countries. Although rates of frank dislocation are lower with universal screening, dislocations are still seen. Higher treatment rates due to the high levels of minor abnormalities picked up by this technique are also considered a problem. A normal screening ultrasound at 6 weeks does not guarantee a normal hip in later life.

At present, there is insufficient evidence to allow clear recommendations on how this should be carried out. According to NIPE guidelines, neonates with risk factors of a positive family history or breech are considered for a hip ultrasound at around 6 weeks of age. Those with positive clinical findings on examination should have an ultrasound performed ideally within 2 weeks. Note that due to ossification of the femoral head that occurs around 4–6 months of age, ultrasound no longer remains an appropriate form of imaging for the hip and plain radiographs become the most appropriate form of imaging.

---

### POINTS TO REMEMBER

1. The Barlow and Ortolani tests are appropriate in those under 3 months of age.
2. Limited hip abduction is a very useful clinical sign of hip dislocation in all ages.
3. Asymmetric thigh creases are sensitive for DDH but in most cases is a normal variant.
4. Ultrasound is considered for at-risk births or those with positive clinical findings.

## Perthes disease

Legg–Calve–Perthes disease is the most common hip disease likely to be encountered. Affecting predominantly males, it occurs within the 4–8 years of age range although not exclusively. Perthes often presents as an acute limp. Parents will often describe a preceding injury or symptoms following excessive activity. The symptoms arise from osteonecrosis of the femoral head. The disease process follows a set of characteristic radiological and clinical stages. The femoral head softens as the body responds to necrotic bone, creating pain and deformity of the hip joint. The blood supply is restored over a period of years. Symptoms are aggravated by physical activity, and most cases will have symptoms that persist with intermittent periods where pain and limp are limited.

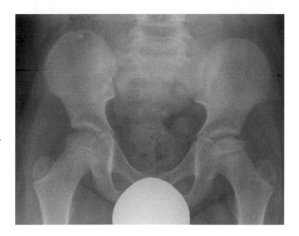

Figure 1.27  Left hip Perthes disease. Note the asymmetry of the femoral epiphysis.

## What is the clinical presentation of perthes disease?

Signs of Perthes disease on examination include an antalgic gait, loss of hip abduction and, in particular, reduced rotation in hip flexion. Some patients will present just with knee pain or thigh pain creating more diagnostic difficulty. The disease process differs in each case with some more severely affected than others. In the initial phases, radiographs may be normal to even trained eyes. As the disease progresses, more classical radiological features such as loss of epiphyseal height and head fragmentation are seen (Figure 1.27). This diagnosis should be considered in any persistent limp in an otherwise well child. It differs from transient synovitis in the persistence of symptoms beyond 1 or 2 weeks.

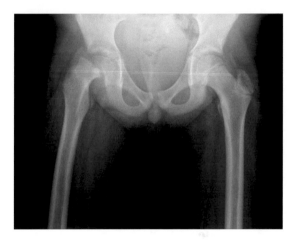

Figure 1.28  Right slipped capital femoral epiphysis (SCFE).

---

### POINTS TO REMEMBER

1. A limping child (aged 4–6 years) with hip pain, persisting for more than 2 weeks, should be examined and investigated to rule out Perthes disease.

## What is SCFE?

A predominately adolescent hip disease, SCFE is rare and a condition where delay in diagnosis is commonly seen following presentation to primary care. The rarity of this disorder means it is unlikely to be seen more than once or twice in a career. The sequelae of late diagnosis have significant implications for the child. Once again, knee pain alone may be the only complaint. The exact pathology of this disorder is unknown. The proximal femoral physis weakens causing the femoral metaphysis to 'slip' leading to deformity and altered mechanics of the hip joint (Figure 1.28).

## What are the clinical manifestations of SCFE?

This condition can present acutely, or as a gradual, chronic process. Chronic slips are more likely to present to primary care as a cause of hip or knee pain associated with a limp. The gait pattern may be antalgic, but a Trendelenburg gait may be seen. Acute slips cause less diagnostic difficulty due to the severity of symptoms. Historically cases were seen more in adolescent boys than girls, although the incidence in females continues to increase. There is an association with obesity. As with Perthes disease, there can be a report of a minor trauma or sports injury after which symptoms began, suggesting a minor groin strain. On clinical examination, hip internal rotation in flexion will be limited, and in more severe slips when the hip is flexed, the leg will turn towards the midline. This is termed obligate external rotation and occurs due to a significant slip of the femoral head.

The key element in diagnosing this condition is the awareness it exists. Early referral for suspected cases is recommended, and in addition, radiographs can identify the diagnosis in all but the mildest of slips.

## POINTS TO REMEMBER

1. An adolescent presenting with hip or knee pain should be examined and investigated for SCFE.
2. Child in the adolescent age presenting with knee pain should have a hip examination and, if necessary, hip x-rays to rule out SCFE.

## What is a toddler's fracture?

These injuries occur around the time of independent walking. A minor trip or fall that may or may not be witnessed results in an inability to weight-bear on one side. This injury normally represents a torsional fracture of the distal tibia. Pain normally settles quickly with immobilisation. Clinically, tenderness may be elicited on palpation of the tibial shaft distally. Toddler's fractures can also occur in the os calcis and lesser bones of the foot, although these are relatively rare.

## POINTS TO REMEMBER

1. There are many causes for a limping child. A thorough history and a detailed examination are necessary to elicit the cause.
2. Any child (especially in the adolescent age) presenting with knee pain should have a hip examination and, if necessary, hip x-rays to rule out SCFE.

## What are the causes of limp in a child?

The cause of a child presenting to primary care with a limp may initially seem difficult to differentiate, but adhering to a set of basic principles in assessment will aid in timely and correct diagnosis. The type of pathology that can be suspected will vary based on the age, chronicity and history of the presenting complaint. It is important to note that 'growing pains' do not present with a limp, and that a potentially treatable condition will be missed if this is assumed. Examination of a child with a limp is critical, and if one point is gained from reading this chapter, it should be that knee pain can be caused by hip pathology as well as knee pathology. The sensory innervation to the knee comes from branches of the obturator nerve which in addition innervates the hip. As a result, a pure hip disorder may present just with knee pain. Younger children can rarely identify the source of pain as the communication skills necessary to relay this are not available to them. A large number of paediatric orthopaedic disorders present with such rarity to general practice that often delays in treatment occur due to misdiagnosis and the difficulty in examination.

## How do you clinically assess a limping child?

### Gait assessment

The limited time available for the examination of patients in primary care means this is often missed, but valuable information can be gained from watching a child walk across the room, even to the inexperienced examiner. Always start with the child's gait when examining. Inability to weight-bear implies pathology that will require an urgent specialist opinion.

Different disorders will cause different types of limp. The patterns are not different from those seen in adults with pathology. The commonest pattern seen in children is the antalgic gait. This implies a short-stepped gait in an attempt to limit spending time on a painful limb, and as a response, more time is spent between steps on the unaffected side. This implies inflammation and can arise from problems in the hip, knee or foot as well as anywhere in the tibia and femur. The Trendelenburg gait results from hip abductor weakness that is unable to maintain pelvic alignment during walking. It is seen in conditions affecting the hip such as Perthes disease, SCFE and DDH. The pelvis will lean away from the affected side to compensate for this weakness.

A short-limbed gait will be seen in limb length discrepancies, and may be the initial presentation of a dislocated hip or congenital limb deficiency. Due to the shortness of a limb, when weight-bearing during walking, the toes on the affected side come in contact with the ground, and will differ from the other side. This must be differentiated from neuromuscular disorders such as cerebral palsy where spasticity leads to toe walking, differing only in the degree of extension of the knee due to the absence of a difference in leg lengths. Unilateral toe walking is sometimes seen in heel pain in children, the commonest cause of which is Sever's disease. Unilateral toe walking is always pathological.

Another important but rare condition to recognise at this stage is muscular dystrophy – a cause of limping in older children. A simple test to perform is observation of a child standing from a floor-sitting position. Due to proximal muscle weakness, the child will use his or her hands to 'walk up' his or her legs in compensation for this weakness. Named Gowers' sign, this, if positive, warrants immediate referral to secondary care.

### Leg length assessment

Another cause of a short-limbed gait, limb length discrepancy, is very difficult to assess accurately, and can easily be incorrectly measured. This is often performed supine on a couch, but it is important to note that even a small degree of tilt of the pelvis will lead to a difference in leg lengths. The easiest way to assess for a difference is with the patient standing with the feet pointing forward. Ensure the knees are straight and the feet flat to the floor. The reference point for assessing a difference is the anterior superior iliac spine. In order to identify this, the examiner should palpate with both thumbs from distal to proximal, stopping at the point prominence when this landmark is reached.

### Hip and knee examination

Key findings in many pathological hip conditions in children manifest with subtle differences in each side on examination. For example, in Perthes disease, the earliest loss of movement is reduced internal rotation of the hip in flexion followed by abduction. In SCFE, again, loss of rotation in flexion may be the only early sign.

## Pyrexia

If febrile and unable to weight-bear, an urgent secondary care opinion is required as there is potential for this to represent septic arthritis or osteomyelitis. Differentiating between active infection and transient synovitis (irritable hip) can be difficult without further investigations. Transient synovitis is probably the most common cause of a limp in the age bracket of 3–8 years. A viral upper respiratory tract infection often predates the onset of the limp but not always. Although children have a painful limp, they tend to be clinically well, with pyrexia less than 38°C. Symptoms settle over 1–2 weeks without long-term sequelae. Clinically, movements of the hip are only slightly limited.

Septic arthritis, osteomyelitis and other infections around the hip such as pyomyositis tend to be associated with a higher degree of pyrexia, in a child who appears unwell. The affected limb will be a lot more irritable and often even limited weight-bearing is painful. Pseudoparalysis is a term often used to describe the attitude of the limb, where the child is reluctant to move the limb, or allow it to be moved. At this point, the infection will be at an advanced stage. Erythema is sometimes seen around the joint although more commonly, there will be warmth that differs to the opposite side. Septic arthritis differs from osteomyelitis in that the presence of sepsis within a joint cavity produces a more dramatic set of clinical signs and general malaise. Often a case of septic arthritis will occur following passage from the metaphysis into the joint cavity. The sequelae of septic arthritis are more significant, as the inflammatory response can rapidly destroy articular cartilage, and from a surgical point of view, these require urgent wash-out. Modern management of osteomyelitis differs in that treatment is nearly always with antibiotic unless there is an intraosseous or periosteal abscess.

## Discitis

Although uncommon, children present in the walking age group with reluctance to weight-bear but normal examination of the lower limbs, often without pyrexia. It is a differential of the younger limping child which is often not considered. Spinal movement such as leaning forwards to pick up an object will be noted to be limited.

---

### POINTS TO REMEMBER

1. The cause of limping changes according to the age of the child.
2. Knee pain and thigh pain can be a sign of hip pathology.
3. Unilateral toe walking is pathological.

---

## Paediatric upper limb problems

What common paediatric problems in the upper limb would one see in the general practitioner (GP) surgery?

Some of common upper limb conditions in a child observed in the GP practice include:

- Trigger thumb
- Camptodactyly
- Clinodactyly
- Polydactyly/syndactyly
- Proximal radioulnar synostosis

## What is congenital trigger thumb?

This presents in infants and toddlers, as a fixed flexion contracture of the interphalangeal joint of the thumb. Often a firm nodule is palpable in the flexor pollicis longus, termed Notta's node. This intrasubstance thickening of the tendon prevents it from tracking through the series of pulleys in the thumb. Often it is noticed after minimal trauma by the parents, where they become aware of the absence of extension in the joint. Many will resolve without a need for surgical intervention. Trigger thumbs in children are not treated with corticosteroid injections seen with adults. Treatment is simple and involves release of the A1 pulley via a small incision at the base of the thumb. Due to the natural history of resolution in many, surgery is deferred until around 18 months of age. Ideally, surgery should be performed before 3–4 years, as joint contractures can develop after this length of time.

---

### POINTS TO REMEMBER

1. Although called a congenital trigger thumb, the flexion deformity is usually absent at birth, and manifests when the child is 6 months old.
2. The condition is generally painless.
3. Surgery is done between 18 months and 4 years of age, depending on the severity.

---

## What is camptodactyly?

A congenital flexion deformity affecting the little finger at the PIP joint, camptodactyly presents either in infancy in males and females or in adolescence mainly in girls. This can be present in different generations of the same family, suggesting an inherited element. It mainly forms a cosmetic problem and, unless the contracture is severe, rarely causes any functional deficit. In severe cases or progressive deformity, splintage is sometimes used. Rarely is surgery indicated (Figure 1.29).

## What is clinodactyly?

This also has a predilection for the little fingers, and is a deformity at the distal interphalangeal

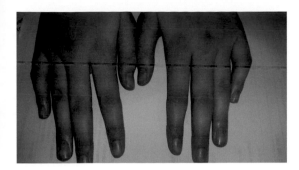

Figure 1.29 Camptodactyly.

joint, with the tip deviated towards or away from the adjacent ring finger in the frontal plane. It is commonly seen in children with Down's syndrome. The deformity often causes concern, but, in most, relatively little functional deficit. As a result, surgery, which can lead to stiffness, is rarely indicated.

## Polydactyly and syndactyly

Polydactyly is divided into preaxial (thumb duplication), postaxial (little finger duplication) or rarely central (index, middle and ring). Syndactyly is described according to the digits involved, and the extent of symphalangism. A simple syndactyly will involve just a skin bridge; a complex may involve shared bone and other tissues. Not all cases will require surgical intervention (Figure 1.30).

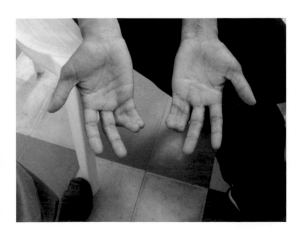

Figure 1.30 Bilateral syndactyly of the fourth and fifth fingers.

## Proximal radioulnar synostosis

This disorder involves a bony or fibrous connection between the proximal radius and ulna, and represents a congenital failure of separation. In roughly half of cases, the condition is bilateral. The result of the synostosis is a loss of forearm rotation. It is often first noted in adolescence, as the ability to compensate for lack of forearm rotation exists due to wrist and shoulder movement. Elbow flexion and extension is rarely involved. Examination of forearm rotation will identify a loss of rotation (Figure 1.31a and b). Excision of the synostosis carries risks of nerve injury and rarely works in restoring rotation. Surgery is limited to rare cases where repositioning the hand by performing a rotational osteotomy through the synostosis will result in better hand placement.

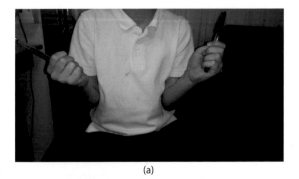

(a)

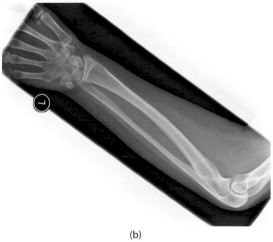

(b)

Figure 1.31 **(a)** Proximal radioulnar synostosis. Note the lack of supination in comparison to the other side. **(b)** Radiograph showing bony synostosis between the proximal radius and ulna.

## Paediatric spine

### What are the causes of back pain in children?

Historically back pain in children has always differed in investigation due to the suggestion that it is rare and always associated with pathology. This statement is not necessarily true, as although less common than in adults, about half of all children by the end of adolescence will have experienced an episode of back pain. The younger the child, the greater the likelihood is of pathology and the need for ongoing review and investigation by both imaging and haematological tests. It is common to have adolescents complain of back pain, and in most cases, this will be related to poor posture associated with modern living. There are conditions such as spondylolysis and Scheuermann's kyphosis that occur mainly in adolescence. Those with hypermobility are also more likely to suffer with back pain. Be aware that a limb length discrepancy can cause both spinal deformity and pain.

### How would you manage back pain in children?

In children, history and examination are most important in differentiating the cause and pattern,

in addition to an understanding of common pathologies seen within each age group. So called 'red flag' symptoms apply both to adults and children. Stiffness may imply an inflammatory arthropathy and constitutional symptoms imply an infection or malignant lesion. Where clinical assessment and symptom patterns raise a low suspicion of pathology, further review is always indicated if it fails to settle. An example of this is back pain after a traumatic injury with minimal symptoms. Haematological investigations including erythrocyte sedimentation rate, C-reactive protein, WBC and rheumatoid factor/anti-nuclear antibodies should be carried out in those that do not fit into this category. If an abnormality is detected and there is a clinical suspicion of an inflammatory arthropathy, a review from a rheumatologist should be obtained. Otherwise, an review by an orthopaedic surgeon should be requested. Plain radiographs rarely help, and MRI is the investigation of choice where no deformity is identified clinically. Most patients benefit from review by a physiotherapist, and often referrals will be recommended by therapists if symptoms do not resolve with their input (Figure 1.32).

### What is scoliosis?

Scoliosis is a coronal malalignment of the spine, although in reality, it is a three-dimensional

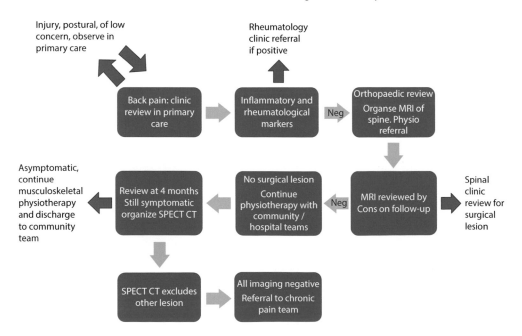

Figure 1.32 Algorithm for management of back pain in children.

deformity associated with rotation of the spine. It is the most common spinal disorder of children and adolescents. It is often divided by onset into infantile (0–3 years), juvenile (4–10 years) and adolescent (11–18 years) as well as according to the pathology (idiopathic or congenital). It is more common in adolescents and females.

## How would you assess a spinal deformity in a child?

Clinical features of spinal deformity are best assessed with a standing patient and suitable clothing to allow assessment of the posterior iliac crests, shoulders and spine. The examination begins with identification of the clinical features that cause patients to present to the surgery. Shoulder asymmetry is noted by many, and gives an idea as to the location of the curve. A prominent rib hump may also be seen. There may also be pelvic tilt, and with a significant fixed curve, the trunk may appear shifted over from the pelvis. From the front, in female patients, breast asymmetry may also be a feature. A postural scoliosis may be present if there is a limb length discrepancy, so it is important this is excluded.

In assessing the degree of a fixed scoliosis, the best way to assess the location and degree of the curve clinically is to perform the Adam's forward bend test. This simple test involves standing behind the patients, asking them to lean forward keeping the knees straight. This will remove any postural element to a scoliosis.

Many cases of scoliosis will have associated intraspinal pathology such as a syrinx or cord tether, so neurological examination is important. Scoliosis can present at different ages depending on the cause. The common types of scoliosis in children are congenital scoliosis and idiopathic scoliosis.

## What is congenital scoliosis?

Congenital scoliosis can be caused by a segmental defects or failure of formation. These tend to present in infancy or childhood, and arise due to the presence or absence of normal elements. The most common findings are either a hemivertebra, or presence of a block vertebra leading to progressive deformity. Although rare, these should be suspected in all young children with fixed spinal deformity, as the natural history is for progression with growth (Figure 1.33).

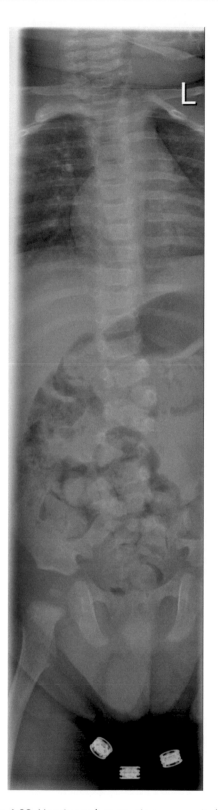

Figure 1.33 Hemivertebra causing congenital scoliosis.

## What is idiopathic scoliosis?

This occurs most commonly in adolescents, although idiopathic cases do occur in juveniles. Adolescent idiopathic scoliosis presents between 10 years of age and skeletal maturity. Age is an important factor, as the younger the patient, the more the growth potential remains for the deformity to progress. The cause is not described although there are genetic factors as demonstrated by twin concordance and familial associations. Early mild deformities can be managed with bracing, although for more severe deformities, spinal surgery is sometimes required (Figures 1.34 and 1.35).

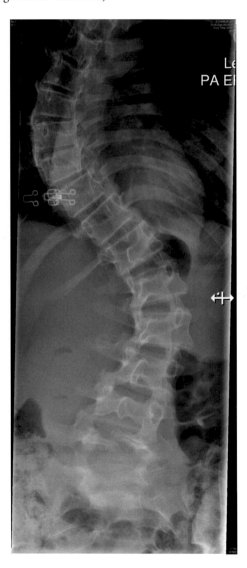

Figure 1.34 Radiograph of adolescent idiopathic scoliosis.

---

**POINTS TO REMEMBER**

1. Scoliosis presents at different ages in children.
2. The nomenclature of the curve is determined by the direction of its convexity.
3. Left dorsal curves especially in idiopathic scoliosis need a neurological assessment as they may be associated with underlying spinal dysraphism.

## What are the other spinal deformities in children, other than scoliosis?

The other deformities include kyphosis (forward bending of spine) and lordosis.

## What is Scheuermann's kyphosis?

Kyphosis (round back deformity) refers to deformity in the sagittal plane. Scheuermann is thought

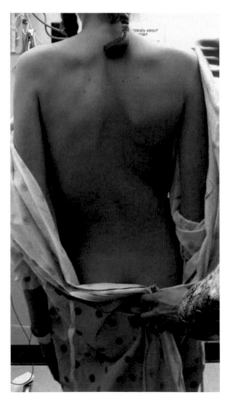

Figure 1.35 Adolescent idiopathic scoliosis. Note the right-sided curve associated with shoulder asymmetry.

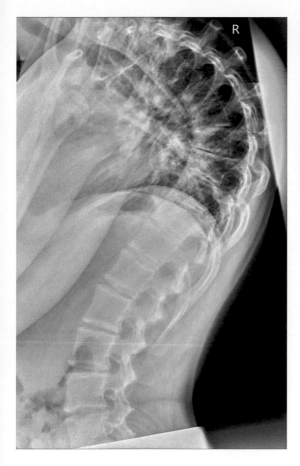

Figure 1.36 Radiograph of Scheuermann's kyphosis.

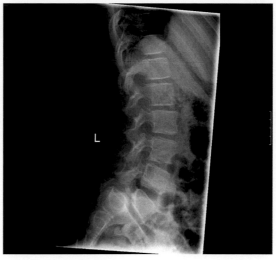

Figure 1.37 Radiograph of a severe spondylolisthesis at the L5/S1 level.

to represent an apophysitis of the vertebral body end plates leading to the development of wedging and subsequent kyphosis. Pain often results at the apex of the deformity. The diagnosis is made radiologically and is dependent on the presence of wedging of three consecutive vertebrae with characteristic end-plate changes. Cases present with pain and deformity. It must be differentiated from postural kyphosis. In cases of Scheuermann's kyphosis, performing an Adam's forward bend test will lead to an exacerbation of the deformity (Figure 1.36).

## What is spondylolisthesis?

This is defined as the forward slippage of one vertebral body on another. Although the aetiology can differ, the cause is a defect in the pars interarticularis bilaterally, termed spondylolysis. This then leads to the slippage and spondylolisthesis. It is most prevalent in the L5 vertebral body, leading to forwards slippage of L5 on the S1 vertebra. It normally presents as localised lower back pain exacerbated by activity. As the degree of slippage worsens, a hyperlordosis may develop with associated hamstring tightness. Neurological signs associated with the S1 or L5 nerve root may also develop. In most cases, any neurological deficit happens gradually as opposed to acutely (Figure 1.37).

Spondylolysis is managed initially with non-operative measures, and can be treated surgically if this fails to control the symptoms of pain. Treatment of listhesis involves fixation in situ.

---

### POINTS TO REMEMBER

1. Scoliosis is the most common form of spinal disorder in children.
2. The progression of the deformity is dependent on age.
3. Back pain in children is common, and the younger the child, the more likely the pathology is present.
4. Postural kyphosis is common but exclude Scheuermann's kyphosis.

## SUMMARY

A large proportion of paediatric orthopaedic problems seen in primary care are physiological and are referred to as normal variants. Most of these correct spontaneously with time. Parental reassurance forms the mainstay of their treatment. A good history from the parents and a thorough clinical examination are imperative to differentiate them from pathological conditions needing active timely intervention. Both the normal variants and pathological conditions have been highlighted in the chapter.

## Suggested Reading

1. Herring JA (ed).*Tachdjian's Paediatric Orthopaedics: From the Texas Scottish Rite Hospital for Children,* 5th Edition. Philadelphia, PA: Elsevier/Saunders, 2014.
2. Jones S, Khandekar S, Tolessa E. Normal variants of the lower limbs in paediatric orthopaedics. *Int J Clin Med.* 2013;4:12–17.
3. Staheli LT. *Fundamentals of Paediatric Orthopaedics.* Philadelphia, PA: Lippincott Williams & Wilkins, 2008.

# 2

# Spine disorders

JASON BRAYBROOKE

## Introduction

Patients with back pain can be one of the most challenging groups of patients to deal with. The majority will have mechanical problems related to posture and aging of the spine – disc dehydration and bulging, and facet joint osteoarthritis, and yet, we are all fearful not to miss the occasional patient who has a more serious underlying cause such as cancer, cauda equina syndrome or progressive neurological deficit.

The burden of back pain in this country is huge – 50% of the UK population report lower back pain for at least 24 hours in any 1 year; half of these report it lasting for 4 weeks and a third for a year. Eighty percent of the population in the United Kingdom will experience back pain in their lifetime; therefore this is the norm and if you never suffer from back pain you are the minority and are abnormal!

How we manage back pain in its early stages affects the outcome – a person who has been on sick leave for 6 months has a 50% chance of returning to work; a person who has been on sick leave for 1 year has a 5% chance of returning to work.

# Back pain

## What is lower back pain?

Back pain is a common symptom in the UK population. Eighty percent of the UK population will complain of an episode of back pain which lasts for 1 month in their lifetime.

## What are the causes of lower back pain?

Lower back pain is most often mechanical, i.e. exacerbated by activity or loading of the spine relieved by rest. The pain can arise from the disc, the facet joint, the muscles and ligaments or the sacroiliac joint. Regardless of the source, the management is similar. This physical component is also influenced to a greater or lesser extent by psychological and social factors. Attention should be paid to establishing the absence of red flag signs suggestive of a more serious underlying condition, spinal infection or tumour (metastasis).

## Red flag signs

- Age <18 years or >55 years*
- Non-mechanical pain
- Night pain
- Thoracic pain
- Use of steroids ≥3 months/drug abuser
- Systemic symptoms of weight loss, night sweats and rigors
- Widespread neurology
- Previous history of cancer/infection
- History of trauma

## What is the natural history of mechanical back pain?

Physical mechanical back pain usually settles in 90% of people within 6–8 weeks. However, if influenced by psychological and social factors it can become chronic (yellow flag):

- Fear avoidance
- Attitudes and beliefs

---

* The red flag sign which is most discriminatory is previous history of cancer/infection and the least discriminatory is age.

- Compensation issues
- Workplace problems
- Family and carers problems

## How to diagnose mechanical back pain

*History (important points)*

- Lower back pain, no radiation below the knee

*Examination (salient features)*

- Restricted range of movement in lumbar spine
- Pain worse on flexion – disc problem
- Pain worse on extension – facetal problem
- Sacroiliac joint stress test – FABER test

FABER test

Figure 2.1 shows the FABER test.

*Treatment options*
Physical component:

- Resume normal activities as soon as possible
- Physiotherapy – postural exercises: facetal flexion exercises, disc extension exercises
- Massage in conjunction with physiotherapy
- Acupuncture
- Transcutaneous electrical nerve stimulation (TENS) machine

Psychological and social component:

- Psychologist: fear avoidance, post-traumatic stress
- Other specialists: RELATE, Department of Work and Pensions (DWP)

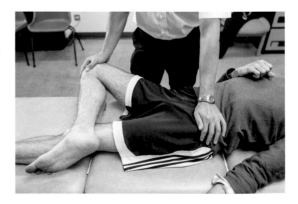

Figure 2.1 FABER's test (Flexion, ABduction and External Rotation).

# Sciatica

## What is sciatica?

Sciatica is a symptom. It is the radiation of pain from the back down the leg which characteristically descends below the knee. It is caused by compression of the nerve roots which contribute to the sciatic nerve (lower lumbar L4, L5 and S1) or femoral nerve (higher lumbar L2 and L3). The pain classically passes down the leg taking a different path for each nerve root affected as below:

L4: Anterior thigh, anterior knee and anteromedial lower leg
L5: Lateral thigh, lateral calf, dorsum of foot and great toe
S1: Buttock, posterior thigh, posterior calf, heel, sole and lateral border of foot

## What is the cause of sciatica?

The most common cause of sciatica is a prolapsed intervertebral disc in 30- to 50–year-olds and foraminal stenosis/narrowing of the exit channel for the nerve root secondary to osteoarthritis in those aged over 65 years.

## What is the natural history of sciatica?

The natural history of sciatica is that in 90% of people, symptoms will improve within 6–8 weeks.

## How to diagnose sciatica

*History (important points)*

- Pain which radiates below the knee
- Associated with pins and needles or numbness/weakness
- Exclude altered urinary or bowel symptoms

*Examination (salient features)*

- Nerve tension signs sequence

1. Straight leg raise (passive test) – increases tension on sciatic nerve, sciatica exacerbated (Figure 2.2)
2. Lasègue test – increases tension on sciatic nerve, sciatica exacerbated (Figure 2.3)
3. Flex knee – relieves tension on sciatic nerve, sciatica settles (Figure 2.4)
4. Femoral stretch test – exacerbates femoratica (Figure 2.5)

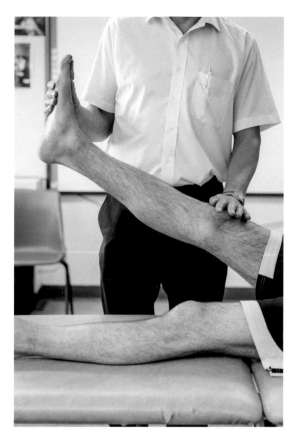

Figure 2.2 Nerve tension sign 1 – straight leg raise.

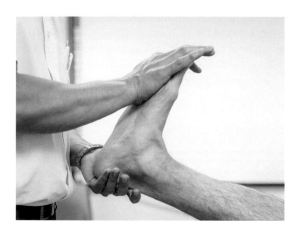

Figure 2.3 Nerve tension sign 2 – Lasegue test.

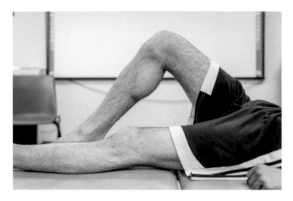

Figure 2.4 Nerve tension sign 3 – flexion of the knee.

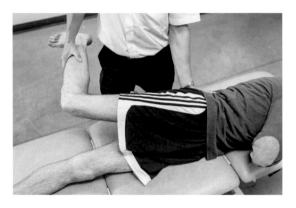

Figure 2.5 Nerve tension sign 4 – femoral stretch test.

*Treatment options*

- Early: NSAIDs, opiates, diazepam, neuropathic agent (gabapentin, pregabalin, amitriptyline), gentle physiotherapy when pain settling
- Transforaminal epidural if the sciatica fails to respond to medication
- Surgery if the sciatica fails to follow its natural history: discectomy – micro-discectomy (with microscope) and mini discectomy (without microscope, no difference in outcomes)

## Cauda equina syndrome

## What is cauda equina syndrome?

Cauda equina syndrome is a condition in which the lumbar and sacral nerve roots (cauda equina) are compressed in the lumbar canal, i.e. below the level of the spinal cord.

## What is the cause of cauda equina syndrome?

Cauda equina syndrome is caused by a large central disc prolapse. It classically presents in 30- to 50–year-olds and has a higher incidence in those people with a higher BMI. It usually presents with crescendo back pain and then perianal numbness and sphincter disturbance.

## What is the natural history of cauda equina syndrome?

The natural history of cauda equina syndrome is that an emergency surgical decompression needs to be performed within 48 hours or ideally within 24 hours of the development of sphincter disturbance (urinary retention/incontinence or faecal incontinence) to recover normal sphincter function.

## How to diagnose cauda equina syndrome

*History (important points)*

- Bilateral sciatica
- Perianal numbness
- Urinary retention/incontinence (frank incontinence not urge or stress incontinence)
- Faecal incontinence

*Examination (salient features)*

- Bilateral straight leg raise positive
- Bilateral neurological foot drops
- Decreased perianal sensation
- Decreased anal tone

*Treatment options*

- Emergency surgical decompression
- Late presentation: leads to a poor outcome which affects quality of life in a young population – sexual dysfunction, bowel regime, intermittent self-catheterisation

## Neurogenic claudication

## What is neurogenic claudication?

Neurogenic claudication is a symptom. The patients describe pain in their legs when they walk.

# What is the cause of neurogenic claudication?

The cause of claudication is either vascular (peripheral vascular disease) or central narrowing of the lumbar canal (lumbar canal stenosis). In vascular claudication, the patient describes pain which starts distally (calves) and radiates proximally. In neurogenic claudication, the patient describes pain which starts proximally and radiates distally. Neurogenic claudication often occurs in people aged over 65 years as it is caused by osteoarthritis in the spine causing compression of the nerve roots. A second peak does occur in a younger age group secondary to congenital narrowing of the lumbar canal. The other cause for neurogenic claudication classically in middle-aged women is a degenerative spondylolisthesis.

# What is the natural history of neurogenic claudication?

Neurogenic claudication is likely to remain static in 70% of people, deteriorates in 15% and improves in 15%.

# How to diagnose claudication

*History (important points)*

- There is restricted walking distance. Patient can walk further using shopping trolley or cycle further than can walk.
- Patients describe that 'legs feel like jelly'.
- They have to sit for 15 minutes to relieve symptoms.

*Examination (salient features)*

- There is usually no abnormal finding other than loss of lumbar lordosis
- Check peripheral pulses to exclude vascular claudication

*Treatment options*

- Conservative: physiotherapy – flexion exercises, exercise bike, neuropathic
- Drugs, nerve root blocks (usually work but don't last long)
- Surgery: decompression of the stenosis lumbar levels

# Brachialgia

## What is brachialgia?

Brachialgia is pain which radiates down the arm characteristically below the elbow, which is caused by compression of the cervical nerve roots C5–T1. The most common nerve roots affected are C6, C7.

## What is the cause of brachialgia?

The most common cause of brachialgia is a prolapsed intervertebral disc in 30- to 50-year-olds and foraminal/lateral recess stenosis secondary to osteoarthritis in those aged over 65 years.

## What is the natural history of brachialgia?

The natural history of brachialgia is very similar to sciatica; it settles down in 90% of people in 6–8 weeks.

## How to diagnose brachialgia

*History (important points)*

- Pain radiates below the elbow
- Paraesthesia
- Head movements exacerbate arm pain/pins and needles

*Examination (salient features)*

- Nerve tension signs – Spurling's test is positive (see below)
- Loss of reflexes
- Dermatomal loss in sensation

**Spurling's test** – With arm and neck extended, lateral flexion and axial pressure on head lead to radiation of pain distally in corresponding dermatome (Figure 2.6).

*Treatment options*

- Early: NSAIDs, opiates, diazepam, neuropathic agent, gentle physiotherapy when settling
- Cervical nerve root block if brachialgia fails to respond
- Surgery: anterior cervical decompression and fusion if brachialgia fails to respond

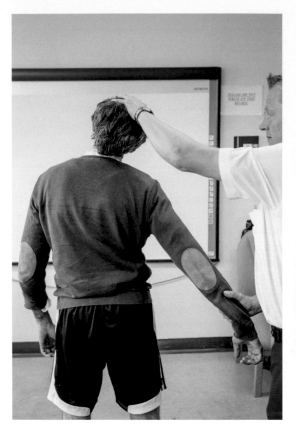

Figure 2.6 Spurling's sign.

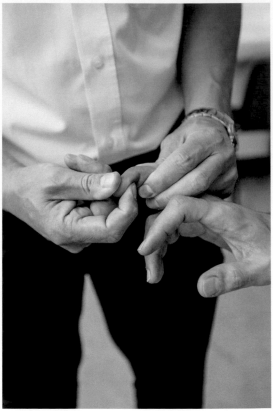

Figure 2.7 Hoffman's sign.

## Cervical myelopathy

### What is cervical myelopathy?

Cervical myelopathy is a condition which develops usually in people aged over 65 years. It is the result of compression of the cervical spinal cord.

### What is the cause of cervical myelopathy?

The cause of cervical myelopathy is usually osteoarthritis of the cervical spine which narrows the cervical spinal canal.

### What is the natural history of cervical myelopathy?

Cervical myelopathy gradually deteriorates in a stepwise fashion. If the patient is symptomatic, the only option is surgery, decompression of the cervical spinal cord.

### How to diagnose cervical myelopathy

*History (important points)*

- Loss of fine motor movement (doing up buttons, knife and fork, writing)
- Stagger like drunk

*Examination (salient features)*

- Spastic gait
- Upper motor neurone signs
- Hoffman's test positive (see below)

**Hoffman's test** – Sudden extension of middle finger leads to flexion of interphalangeal joint (IPJ) of thumb and distal interphalangeal joint (DIPJ) of index finger (Figure 2.7).

*Treatment options*

Surgical decompression of the cervical spinal cord can be considered to guarantee no progression of disease. However, this does not necessarily mean recovery of symptoms.

---

## SUMMARY

1. The majority of back and neck pain is mechanical and benign. The natural history is influenced by psychosocial factors.
2. Red flag signs are useful to determine those patients with more serious underlying pathology.
3. If the neurological deficit can be explained by a single nerve root, this is reassuring and the prognosis in the majority (90%) will be good.

## Resources

1. BackCare – www.backcare.org.uk
2. BASS – British Association of Spine Surgeons – www.spinesurgeon.ac.uk
3. Arthritis Research UK – www.arthritisresearchuk.org

## Suggested Reading

1. Palmer KT, Walsh K, Bendall H, Cooper C, Coggon D. Back pain in Britain: Comparison of two prevalence surveys at an interval of 10 years. *BMJ*. 2000;320:1577–1578.
2. Maniadakis A, Gray A. The economic burden of back pain in the UK. *Pain*. 2000;84:95–103.
3. Department of Health. *The Prevalence of Back Pain in Great Britain in 1998*. London: Department of Health, 1999.
4. Waddell G, McIntosh A, Hutchinson A, Feder G, Lewis M. *Low Back Pain Evidence Review*. London: Royal College of General Practitioners, 1999.

# Shoulder disorders

## ALISON ARMSTRONG

## Introduction

The purpose of the shoulder joint is to position the hand in space. It has a very wide range of movement through half a circle in several directions and trades stability for mobility. In fact, it is not one joint but four: two true joints and two 'pseudo-joints'. In assessing a patient with a shoulder disorder, the history and examination need to separate out these four joints. This arguably makes the examination of the shoulder more complex than other joints and it has thus acquired the reputation of being 'unfathomable'. Through this chapter, I hope to demystify the diagnosis of shoulder problems and their management.

## Some key principles to get started

1. *Number of joints/pseudo-joints*
   There are two joints (glenohumeral and acromioclavicular [AC]) and two 'pseudo-joints' (the subacromial space and scapulothoracic space), and the examination needs to separate those out.
2. *Separate out shoulder pain from neck pain*
   Pain in the shoulder may come from the neck and needs to be differentiated right at the start (neck and shoulder pain may coexist).
3. *The shoulder joint has little intrinsic stability*
   The glenohumeral joint has no intrinsic stability, part of the trade-off for a very large range of movement. It has been described as a ball on

a vertical plate and it depends on the muscles and capsule around it to keep it in the joint and moving properly. Instability and muscle incoordination are therefore not uncommon, particularly in the young and lax.

4. *Muscle function and control are important because of a lack of bony stability*
The only bony contact between the hand and the chest wall is through the sternoclavicular joint. This means that the whole of the shoulder girdle relies on a well-functioning scapular musculature. If the muscles are poorly coordinated, or coping with another group of muscles that are not functioning properly, then the scapula may not move correctly and will become painful.

5. *Shoulder disease groups*
Diseases of the shoulder fall into four categories:
   a. Dislocation: stretching of the capsule or damage to the disc around the glenoid
   b. Wear:
      i. Of the joints giving rise to arthritis
      ii. Of the tendons of the rotator cuff
   c. Neurological injury
   d. Infection/tumour

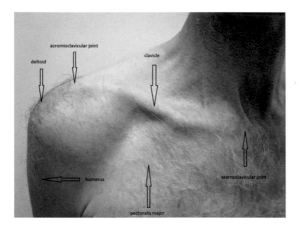

Figure 3.1　Important surface anatomical landmarks.

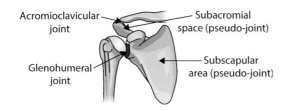

Figure 3.2 Bony anatomy of the shoulder showing joints (2) and pseudo-joints (2).

## Anatomy of the shoulder

1. Important surface anatomy (Figure 3.1)
2. Four 'joints' (Figure 3.2)
3. Muscle groups (Figure 3.3)
4. Bursae of shoulder (Figure 3.4)

## Initial assessment

1. How do patients present?
Patients are likely to present with one of three problems alone or in combination:

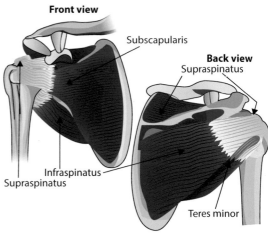

Figure 3.3　Muscles of the rotator cuff.

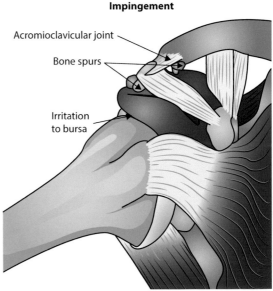

Figure 3.4　Subacromial bursa of shoulder.

a. Pain
b. Instability
c. Lump
2. What questions should I ask?
There are six important questions to ask:
   a. What are the symptoms?
      Common symptoms: Pain, stiffness, insta-
         bility, weakness
      Rare (could be serious): Lump or swelling
      Pain: An ache or sharp
      Stiffness: In the morning, it just will not
         move, or it can move but patient can-
         not move it
      Instability: Frank dislocation, feeling of
         looseness, feeling of 'a guy rope loose',
         clicks and grinds
      Weakness: Heaviness on lifting the arms,
         dropping things, loss of control on lift-
         ing things, can't do overhead activities
      Lump/swelling: Could be ganglia (from AC
         joint) or lipomata, but may represent
         malignancy
   b. Where is the pain?
      Is it in the neck, shoulder (glenohumeral/
         subacromial), AC, scapular?
      Eliminate the neck from enquiry early (see
         Figure 3.5)
   c. When does the pain come on?
      (Note that night pain may be a reason to
         present, but it isn't diagnostic.)
      Red flag: Night and day, at rest, no relief
         with simple painkillers
      On activity: Most shoulder conditions
   d. Is there a history of trauma or overuse – and
      did the pain start straight away or the next day?
      Red flag: Fall with weakness (acute cuff
         tear), fall with odd-shaped shoulder
         (dislocation), electric shock/fit (unre-
         duced posterior shoulder dislocation),
         fall with severe pain (fracture)
      Pain the next day: Unlikely a cuff tear,
         but could be impingement syndrome,
         frozen shoulder arthritis or muscle
         imbalance (in the young)
      Pain at the time of injury: Think red flag or
         cuff tear
   e. Are there other odd symptoms: paraesthe-
      sia, shooting pains in the arms, numbness?
      Odd neurological type symptoms may
      indicate the neck as the source but can be
      found in frozen shoulder. Brachial neuritis

(weakness of muscles of shoulder typically
supra/infraspinatus, deltoid and biceps)
may start with a rush of pain and, 1 week
later, weakness.
   f. Other medical history
      Diabetes: Think frozen shoulder
      Epilepsy: Think dislocation anterior or
         posterior
      Joint laxity: Think muscle patterning
         problem/instability
      Inflammatory arthritis: All the common
         causes of shoulder pain especially.
         Glenohumeral arthritis and cuff
         weakness/rupture
      Previous malignancy: Think secondaries

## Examination

1. *If the patient gives a history of dislocation*
   The history of the part dislocated will give the
   likely diagnosis. Tests to elucidate the nature
   of the dislocation are beyond the remit of this
   book and usually unnecessary in primary care.
   It may be useful to ascertain if they are generally joint lax by performing the Beighton score
   (scored out of 9, see Table 3.1). A score of 4 or
   over is considered lax jointed.
2. *If the patient gives a history of a painful shoulder*
   Initially, the most important fact to ascertain is
   which of the four groups the painful shoulder
   belongs to. I call it the **4 Ns**.

   a. It's the **neck**
   b. Something **nasty**: infection malignancy
   c. **Not** moving: stiff frozen shoulder, gleno-
      humeral arthritis, posteriorly dislocated
      glenohumeral joint
   d. **Normal** movement but it is painful:
      impingement syndrome (positive or nega-
      tive cuff disease), AC joint arthritis

NB: Impingement syndrome in those aged under
40 years is most likely proprioceptive incoordination until proved otherwise (i.e. poor muscle control or aberrant muscle movements).

1. **Neck**
   It is worth examining the neck first. If moving the neck reproduces the pain, it is a neck
   problem and not the shoulder. The pain in the
   trapezius is from the neck, not the shoulder.
2. **Nasty**
   A severely painful shoulder joint that will
   barely move – think malignancy, infection

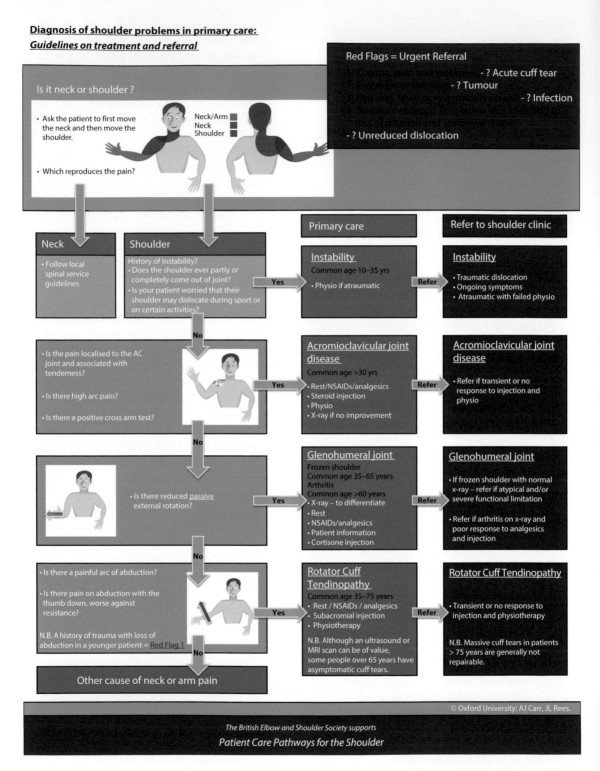

Figure 3.5 Useful algorithm to follow when seeing a patient with Shoulder pain. (From Kulkarni R et al., *Shoulder Elbow*, 2015;7(2):135–143.)

> **Summary of questions to ask about shoulder pain.**
> i) What is the symptom?
> ii) Where is the pain?
> iii) When does the pain come on?
> iv) Trauma or overuse?
> v) Other odd symptoms?
> vi) Other medical conditions?

Table 3.1 Beighton score

**(4 or more = lax)**

1. Little finger hyperextended more than 90° (2 points)
2. Thumb can bend back and reach forearm (2 points)
3. Elbow extension is more than 10° beyond neutral (2 points)
4. Knee extension is more than 10° beyond neutral (2 points)
5. Patient on flexing at hip (knees extended, no shoes worn) can put hands flat on floor (1 point)

*Source:* Beighton P, Horan F, *J Bone Joint Surg [Br]*, 1969;51:444–453.

or acute calcific tendonitis – or in the case of trauma fracture. Calcific tendonitis is not a red flag diagnosis, but the pain of calcific tendonitis (usually because the calcium is leaving the tendon) is extremely painful and can mimic the 'nasty' cases. An x-ray will help in the diagnosis. Note that bilateral morning stiffness suggests polymyalgia rheumatic (PMR).

If you are sure, refer immediately for infection, urgently for cancer.

If you are only suspicious, an x-ray will help with malignancy, fracture, infection and calcific tendonitis. C-reactive protein (CRP) may help if infection needs to be excluded and to contribute to the diagnosis of PMR.

3. **Not moving**
   This is the group of conditions that causes a stiff shoulder in all directions of movement. They cannot move it fully and neither can you. Usually what they can do themselves is the same as what you achieve, and usually the pain comes on at the end of movement. The easiest movement to check

is external rotation, mainly because elevation in other conditions can be so painful that you cannot achieve this, whereas external rotation with the arm by the side can be achieved.

Passive external rotation is required: do not bother with active movement (if you only do active movement, you will miss the diagnosis). Do compare to the other side. External rotation varies among people from 30° to 100° so an external rotation of 50° is only reduced in someone whose normal rotation is more than this: see Figure 3.6 where normal ER is about 90° and reduced is about 60°.

4. **Normal movement but painful**
   a. Ask the patients to lift their arm up and tell you where it hurts. If halfway up or from halfway, it may be impingement syndrome. If it is up at the top, it may be AC joint arthritis. You can check the AC joint to see if it is sore to touch (Figure 3.7).
   b. Test their power by holding the arm at 30° abduction thumbs down. If it is weak, the cuff may be torn (*note:* if very painful, the cuff may appear weak by pain inhibition). This is sometimes called the 'empty can test' (position of the arm when emptying a can).

## How to manage the shoulder at this stage?

You may find the algorithm in Figure 3.5 helpful in managing the painful shoulder.[1]

1. **Red flags needing urgent referral**
   a. Suspected infection: Emergency same day referral
   b. Suspected fracture: Referral to fracture clinic or A and E

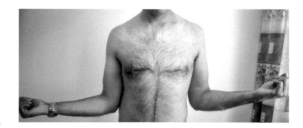

Figure 3.6 Loss of external rotation demonstrated, note on better side External rotation is about 90°.

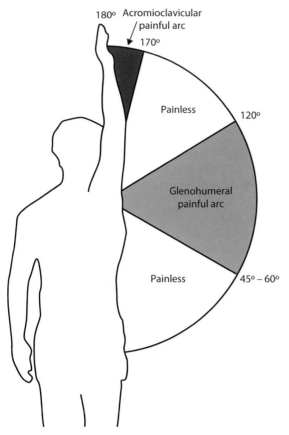

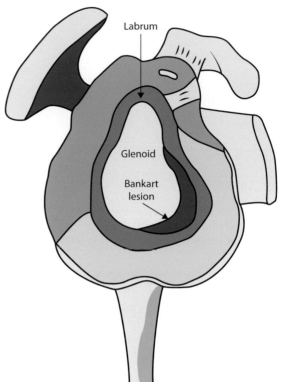

Figure 3.7 Demonstration of painful arcs in shoulder. Mid arc (sub acromial), high (acromioclavicular).

Figure 3.8 Specimen, looking at glenoid. To show labrum (fibrous disc around glenoid) pulled off in traumatic dislocation.

c. Suspected malignancy: Follow 2-week cancer referral pathway
d. Unreduced dislocation: Emergency referral same day
e. Acute cuff tear secondary to trauma: Urgent referral to fracture clinic according to local guidelines
2. For other conditions see next section.

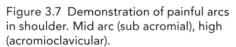

| Examination | Red flags need referral urgent/ immediately |
|---|---|
| a. Is it the neck? | |
| b. Is it something nasty? | a. Infection |
| c. Not normal movement? | b. Fracture |
| | c. Malignancy |
| d. Normal movement but pain? | d. Unreduced dislocation |
| | e. Acute cuff tear |

## Conditions in more detail

## Dislocating shoulder (glenohumeral joint)

1. *What is the reason a shoulder dislocates?*
   There are essentially two types of dislocations. Patients are typically aged 10–35 years.
   a. Those that happen without injury in the lax jointed (high Beighton score) . Typically, the capsule is stretched (see Figure 3.9).
   b. Those that happen after trauma in the lax and non-lax jointed. The capsule may be stretched or the fibrous disc around the glenoid may be ripped off (see Figure 3.8).
2. *What do I do with a shoulder that dislocates?*
   Atraumatic dislocations can be referred to a physiotherapy expert in shoulder stabilisation. If they are unsuccessful then refer into secondary care.

Traumatic dislocations will need investigating if the patient wants treatment (whether there is laxity of the joints, as lax-jointed people may still get Bankart lesions). Refer these to secondary care. Those under age 24 years at the time of their first traumatic dislocation are extremely likely to have continuing problems (40-year-olds tend to be a bit stiff, which eases and they are then usually fine. Those who are around 60 years of age will probably have a rotator cuff tear: see below).

a. *What do I discuss with the patient before referral?*
   Surgery is indicated for structural lesion. If there is no structural lesion, then physiotherapy (done by the patient with advice from the physiotherapist) will be required. This involves about 30 minutes per day over a 4–5-month period and can be longer. That means the patients need to be committed to it.

   It is important to establish that the patient wants and is prepared to have treatment before referral.
   Once the dislocation has been reduced, some patients lose interest in any long-term prevention. As stated above, if they are under the age of 24 years, recurrent dislocations are very common. Some, especially the atraumatic dislocators, even make it a 'party trick' and a way of earning money (see Figure 3.9).

## Painful shoulders

1. *Some general principles*
   a. A painful shoulder that is not showing signs of getting better within 3 weeks probably isn't going to heal on its own and will need help. Rest for a few weeks can be helpful, as can nonsteroidal anti-inflammatory drugs (NSAIDs) whilst waiting.
   b. It is always worth re-examining a shoulder, as a frozen shoulder can resolve and an impingement syndrome can get a frozen shoulder added on top.
   c. If referred for physiotherapy and they are not making significant progress within 6 weeks, refer on.

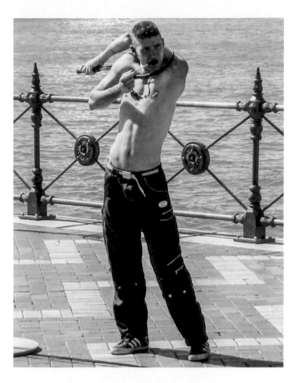

Figure 3.9 Voluntary posterior dislocation of shoulder joint enables a man to pass through a tennis racket.

d. Steroid injections appropriately given to the correct site may help, but more than two in any one area is not recommended. An injection that only gives a month's relief will not give more relief if repeated. Steroid injections are thought to weaken the cuff (though there is no firm evidence for this).

e. Plain x-rays (anteroposterior [AP] and axial) can be useful to separate glenohumeral problems from subacromial space. However, in the presence of glenohumeral arthritis, the source of pain could be from the subacromial space. You should not, therefore, rely on x-ray alone to establish the diagnosis.

f. An ultrasound report may detect partial thickness tears, which may not be symptomatic. Magnetic resonance imaging (MRI) scans are rarely indicated in primary care.

2. *What causes a painful shoulder?*
   From your examination, it should have been possible to eliminate the neck

symptoms. If you are suspicious of malignancy or infection, the patient will need referring. That just leaves the last two categories: not moving (stiff) or normal movement but painful. The causes and management of these will now be discussed.

## Not moving – stiff painful shoulder

1. *What will I find on examination?*
   a. Passive external rotation is reduced compared to the other side.
   b. Active and passive elevation will be reduced to the same amount.
2. *What are the diagnostic possibilities?*
   This is either a frozen shoulder (Figure 3.10) or glenohumeral arthritis (Figure 3.11) or, in rare cases, a red flag: a locked posterior dislocation (see diagram in Figure 3.12 and clinical picture in Figure 3.13a and b).
   • Typically, a frozen shoulder occurs in those aged 35–65 years and it doesn't creak.
   • Typically, a patient with arthritis is aged over 60 years and it may creak (but osteoarthritis [OA] can occur in patients younger than this).
   • In the older patient (in 70s), a frozen shoulder is rare; more common is OA.
   • An x-ray is the only way to distinguish the two. The axial view is usually the most useful.

Frozen shoulder

1. *What is a frozen shoulder?*
   The coracohumeral ligament become contracted. A frozen shoulder classically runs through three stages: freezing, frozen and thawing phases. Each stage typically lasts 4–8 months. The condition may run for 2–3 years, and not everyone recovers. It can be the first sign of a type II diabetes (but mostly not).

   The freezing stage (for some, not all patients) can be very painful, night and day. In the very early stages, it can look like impingement, so it's worth examining for if the patient continues to have pain. A frozen shoulder can sit on top of

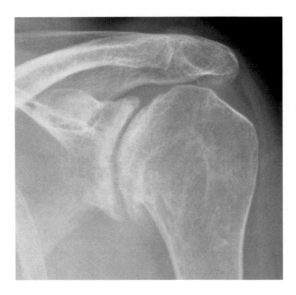

Figure 3.11 Specimen – glenohumeral joint arthritis on x-ray – showing reduced joint space and inferior osteophyte.

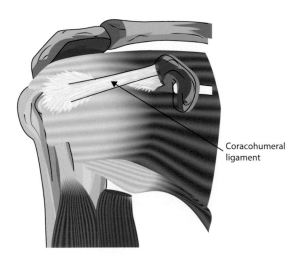

Figure 3.10 Specimen – showing tight coracohumeral ligament in shoulder.

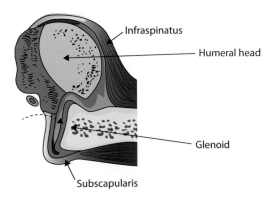

Figure 3.12 Specimen – showing humeral head locked behind the glenoid.

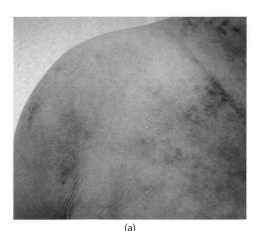

(a)

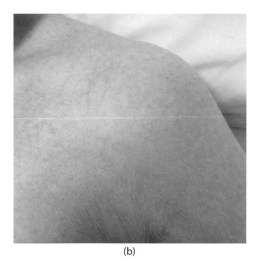

(b)

Figure 3.13 Clinical picture of **(a)** locked posterior dislocation and **(b)** normal other shoulder. Note the dislocated shoulder looks very similar to the normal shoulder (bruising apart).

any painful condition (so it can mask impingement syndrome, which will only appear again when the frozen shoulder is treated). A frozen shoulder can also coexist with a cuff tear.

2. *How is frozen shoulder managed?*
   a. Milder cases can be managed initially with NSAIDs. More severe cases will be helped by a glenohumeral joint injection of steroid and, initially, local anaesthetic to help with the pain, and then a referral to secondary care to get the movement back.
   b. In some circumstances, physiotherapy can be helpful. If the shoulder is very painful,

then the physiotherapy may be counterproductive as the stretching may further inflame the shoulder.
   c. The only investigation that is useful is an x-ray (AP and axial).
   d. Referral to secondary care: in secondary care, the range of shoulder movement can be restored by distension arthrogram, manipulation under anaesthesia (MUA) or arthroscopic interval release. The best method is not currently known and is the subject of a national randomised controlled trial.

3. *What to discuss pre-referral?*
   The patient is likely to need something done (operation/investigation). The treatment options include MUA, distension arthrogram (awake) or key hole surgery. These require a very short stay in hospital which has to be followed by intensive physiotherapy for 2–3 months. Patients can drive and return to work when safe (after 1–2 weeks). The success rate is about 90%. Waiting doesn't make the operation more difficult, nor worsen the outcome, but it does prolong the suffering.

Glenohumeral arthritis

1. *How to manage glenohumeral OA*
   a. The management is the same as for OA anywhere. NSAIDs, lifestyle advice (thinking about job changes or retirement) and eventually joint replacement.
   b. Physiotherapy has a limited role. Steroid injections can help short-term flare-ups. Intra-articular collagen injections may have a limited role for early arthritis (need referral to secondary care for this).
   c. Refer when the pain starts to interfere with their life (and usually sleep).

*What to discuss before referral?*
Joint replacement risks are the same as for other large joints with similar risk ratios. An intact and functioning cuff is required for primary joint replacement. The aim of the operation is pain relief rather than more movement. The best likely movement is 120° of flexion. The in-hospital stay is usually about 3 days, while a sling is required for 3–6 weeks. It takes about 3 months to get over the worst of the operation and about a year to get back to their best. Joint replacement patients are not advised to

continue a job with heavy lifting (so for some early retirement is a consideration).

### Posterior dislocation of the shoulder

1. *What is the presentation?*

   Usually, sudden onset of a painful and restricted range of active and passive movements. This looks exactly like a frozen shoulder or glenohumeral arthritis. Posterior dislocations occur after epileptic fits, road accidents and electric shocks.
   In general practice, you are most likely to come across this with an epileptic fit (often nocturnal).

Causes of stiff shoulders are
- Frozen shoulder
- Glenohumeral joint OA
- Locked posterior dislocation

## Patients who have painful shoulder but normal passive movements

In this group, the key examination finding is that their passive movement is normal compared to the other side. Checking the external rotation is often easiest (should be same on both sides). Cuff power (use the empty can test) may be weak if the cuff is ruptured (but it may just be weak because of the pain).

## Acromio-clavicular (AC) joint pain

### AC joint OA (Figure 3.14)

   This commonly affects people over 30 years of age. The AC joint is palpable and will be sore if affected. It can also cause impingement syndrome as the AC joint swells with reduction in the space for the tendon underneath to glide past.

1. *How to manage the condition*

   The first line of management is a trial of rest and NSAIDs. A steroid injection can be given into the joint, but the landmarks can be difficult to feel, especially in obese people. As such, it is better done under x-ray or ultrasound scan (USS) control. If these measures fail or just give temporary relief, these patients should be referred.

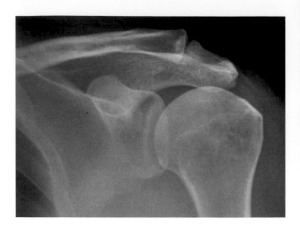

Figure 3.14 X-ray showing enlarged and arthritic acromioclavicular joint.

2. *Pre-referral counselling*

   At operation, the AC joint is excised, and this can be done arthroscopically. It takes about 3 months to recover which means patients may need to be on light activities for this period.

### Osteolysis of distal clavicle

   In rare cases, the symptoms may be due to osteolysis of the distal clavicle. The clavicle resorbs and then reforms over a 2-year period, diagnosed by x-ray. Initial treatment is the same as for OA of the AC joint and generally gets picked up in secondary care. If it doesn't settle with steroid injections, the joint can be excised.

### Disrupted AC joint disc

   Clicking of the AC joint (especially after trauma) can be from disruption of the disc in the joint. The treatment is the same as for OA.

## Impingement syndrome – normal cuff

This is the name given to the collection of diseases with similar findings on x-ray. The current belief is that the tendon (typically supraspinatus; see Figure 3.15) and/or bursa, above the tendon but below the acromion, has too little space to move around. This results in squashing of the tendon in certain positions leading to swelling of the tendon and inflammation of the bursa (see Figure 3.4), which then means there is even less room for the tendon to move around. It is believed that there is a hook at the front of the acromion but it is not known whether the hook develops or was always there (see Figure 3.16).

Typically, this occurs in 40–60-year-olds. It can occur without trauma, or after trauma or repetitive injury.

Beware of this condition when in the under 40s. In these cases, it may be due to poor muscle control around the shoulder (proprioceptive inco-ordination) as opposed to a hook. Often these patients are lax jointed. In this condition, the cuff muscles around the glenohumeral joint do not control the head on the glenoid precisely. Instead, the head may wobble around so that the cuff hits the acromion above with elevation of the arm. These patients need physiotherapy exercises with a shoulder expert, and a steroid injection will be ineffective.

*How to manage patients with impingement syndrome*

1.  Rest the patient to allow the inflammation to settle with NSAIDs (only for about 3 weeks

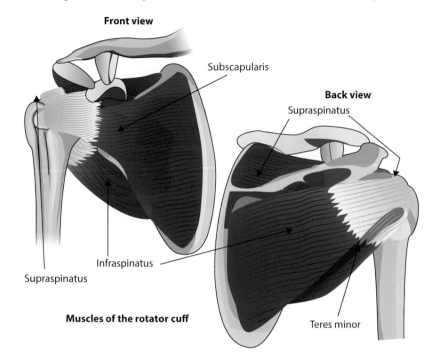

Figure 3.15 Models of shoulder girdle showing muscles and tendons around the shoulder. Tendon that gets compressed in shoulder is usually supraspinatus.

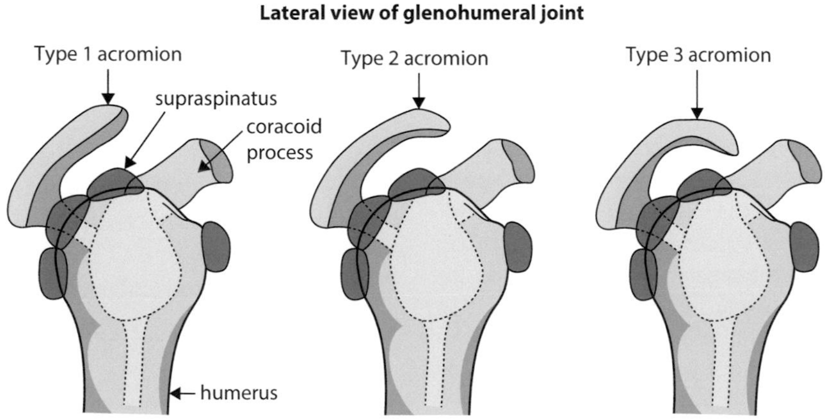

Figure 3.16 Diagrams to show hooks of acromion.

before moving on to other treatments).

2. If there was trauma it may be worth doing an USS, as not all patients with a cuff tear will have weakness (although the majority do).

3. Physiotherapy can be effective (particularly if the AC joint is normal). Exercises may improve the control of the cuff muscles on elevating the shoulder and get rid of the pinching of the tendon.

4. A steroid injection into the subacromial space can reduce inflammation and allow healing. Whether it is effective in the long term will depend on the tightness of the space. This can be effectively combined with physiotherapy.

5. If after resting for 3 weeks with one steroid injection and a course of physiotherapy, the patient is not better, refer to secondary care. It is likely they will need decompression surgery.

### Pre-referral counselling

At operation, a piece of bone at the front of the shoulder is removed to create more space for the tendon to move around (plus/minus the AC joint). This is usually performed by keyhole surgery. Exercises should be started straight away after the surgery. It can be 6 weeks to 3 months before the patient feels better and up to 9 months for them to get back to their best. The patient may need to be excused from heavy lifting for 3 months, and the average return to driving is about 4 weeks.

## Variants

## Calcific tendonitis (Figure 3.17)

### What is calcific tendonitis?

In some people, when the tendon is squashed calcium (calcium hydroxyapatite) is deposited. This may be deposited without symptoms, or else the calcium can resorb or disgorge into the subacromial space. If the calcium disgorges into the space, it is very irritating to the tissue (and may cause sudden intense acute shoulder pain mimicking infection). The initial management is the same as for impingement syndrome, but because the pain is so severe, a swift steroid and local anaesthetic injection may be of help (but you will need to exclude infection, as sometimes it can be a mimic).

If an injection doesn't help, then refer to secondary care.

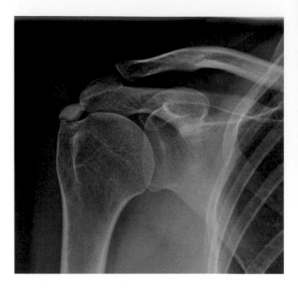

Figure 3.17 X-ray of calcific tendonitis. Note the calcium in the cuff (arrowed).

### Pre-referral counselling

At operation, the surgeon will remove the hook (as above) and may remove the calcium, depending on the size and if it is still there.

Recovery is the same as for impingement syndrome but may be a little slower if calcium is removed. The patient has increased risk of a frozen shoulder postoperatively.

## Cuff tears

This group of patients appear to have impingement syndrome but may have weakness on cuff testing. They Tears of the rotator cuff (see Figure 3.18) may present with a spectrum of clinical syndromes which makes the management more complicated. A common presentation is impingement syndrome with a weak cuff on formal testing but the spectrum includes the following:

- Pseudoparalysis
- A painful arc with weak cuff power
- Normal pain free movement but weakness on formal cuff tearing
- A silent dislocation (elderly massive rotator cuff tear)
- Recurrent dislocation (elderly, massive tears)

There will be patients who have had definite trauma, i.e. a fall, an accident when they knew something went in their shoulder associated

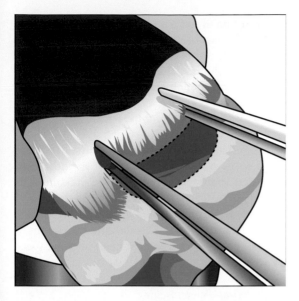

Figure 3.18 Specimen. Cuff tear appearance.

with pain and weakness on cuff testing. These symptoms are red flags and the patient should be referred.

However, not all tears are symptomatic and not all tears are associated with a definite injury. Some tears are only partial. In the group of patients who have degenerate tears, it is reasonable to treat them as if there was no tear and use rest, NSAIDs and physiotherapy and a steroid injection, but with a lower threshold for referral if they do not respond.

Massive cuff tears in those aged over 75 years are rarely repairable. They can respond to a particular form of physiotherapy (the Ainsworth regime) which may be combined with a steroid injection or other pain relief. They may take 4–5 months to get back to their best. They should be referred if this does not help.

### What to watch out for?

In rare cases, without trauma or a week after trauma, there are patients who have a sudden onset of pain followed by weakness. Typically, there are no sensory symptoms but motor weakness affecting deltoid, cuff muscles and biceps. This may be due to brachial neuritis/neuralgic amyotrophy/Parsonage–Turner syndrome. Nerve studies are needed and it is best to refer to secondary care. The management is non-surgical.

### Who to refer?

1. Red flags: acute tear, dislocated or dislocatable. Immediate referral.
2. Those aged under 75 years with short trial (a few months maximum) of conservative management. However, if they are pain-free and have no functional limitation, even if they have a tear, surgery won't usually be offered.
3. Those aged over 75 years if they have pain. There is little that can be done for pseudoparalysis. A painless shoulder with full movement and some weakness above shoulder height does not need surgery.

### Pre-referral counselling

There are a number of options depending on age and tear size, so it is difficult to be prescriptive. We do not always repair the cuff tear. There are other operative procedures such as nerve block (with thermal damage to suprascapular nerve), debridement of tendon, patch repair of the tendon, reverse shoulder replacement and muscle transfer.

In general, repairing the cuff is a big operation. It may take about 4–5 months of physiotherapy and that length of time to get to feel better than preoperatively and up to 18 months to get back to their best. They may be off driving for 8 weeks and off heavy lifting for up to 9 months. Cuff repairs can fail (but are not always symptomatic). Success rates depend on the cuff quality, the size of the tear, the age of the patient, the length of time the tendon has been torn and the muscle quality of the cuff muscles.

---

**Causes of a Painful Shoulder with normal passive movement**
- Acromioclavicular joint pain
- Impingement syndrome
  - with or without cuff tear
  - with or without calcific tendonitis

---

## Scapula

This bone is held in place almost entirely by muscles and control of the muscle pull is important. It is therefore prone to behave abnormally when muscles are poorly controlled.

Typical problems are as follows:

1. **Lumps:** These are a red flag and should be referred.

2. **Clicks at the top of the scapula:** This is usually because the muscles are deranged and have pulled the scapula up and forwards so that the top of the scapula rubs on the ribs. Refer to secondary care for assessment. It is important to exclude bony growth on the underside of the scapula as the cause before referral to physiotherapy. If there is bone growth, it may need excision of superior pole of scapula.

3. **True winging of the scapula:** This is when the patient leans their hands forwards against the door with the elbows straight and shoulder elevated to 90° and the scapula sticks out (see Figure 3.19). The usual cause is a problem relating to the long thoracic nerve resulting in loss of function, of which there are many causes. This needs referral to secondary care.

4. **Pseudo-winging (and scapula** dysrhythmia)**:** When the scapula clearly isn't moving normally but formal winging tests are negative. Usually, this is secondary to muscle incoordination around the shoulder. Specialist assessment is advised, as there are many causes.

> **Causes of Scapula Problems**
> - Poor rhythm (pseudo-winging and dysrhythmia)
> - Clicks
> - Winging

## Steroid injections

Done properly for the correct indications, these can be very helpful. There are three typical places that injection may be of use:

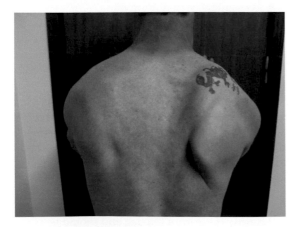

Figure 3.19    Winged right scapula.

1. Subacromial space for impingement syndrome (but not in those aged under 40, or for acute traumatic tears)
2. The glenohumeral joint (for painful frozen shoulder, although not much use if stiff, and for painful OA)
3. The AC joint (for OA of the joint)

It is advised that an injection course is undertaken to gain confidence. One, or at most two, injections should be considered the maximum in primary care. It is only reasonable to do the second injection if there was long-lasting or significant benefit from the first. The absolute maximum is three in one area in a year. When referring, specify which space was injected: do not just say 'the shoulder'.

*Pre-injection counselling*: It may take a week to work or may work temporarily. There is a 1 in 40,000 risk of infection and the patient may get flushing. Anaphylaxis has been described, although it is rare.

## Subacromial injection

- Probably the easiest to undertake
- Either posterior (preferable) or lateral approach

In the posterior approach, the needle goes in at 2 cm medial and inferior to scapula posterior angle. Mark this with the needle cover before cleaning to mark the spot (Figure 3.20a through d).

In obese people, there can be up to 2.5 cm of fat above the acromion so you need to identify the acromial posterior corner and inject under the acromion.

Triamcinolone acetate (40 mg) with 0.5% bupivacaine 9 mL is recommended. The volume is useful to get the steroid around the space.

## Glenohumeral injection

The posterior approach is easiest. Insertion point is as for subacromial injection, head for the tip of the coracoid. This will be more difficult in the obese (Figure 3.21a).

Use the same mixture as for subacromial injection. Mark the skin as before. The injection material should go in quite easily if you are in the joint (Figure 3.21b).

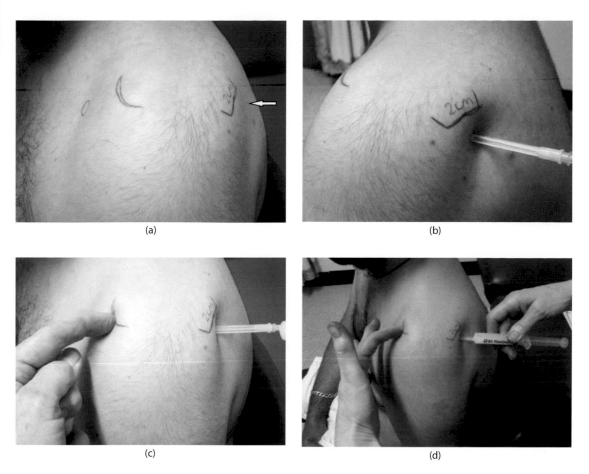

Figure 3.20  Subacromial injection. **(a)** Mark the skin entry point 2 cm medial to the point of the posterior point of the acromion and 2 cm inferior (see arrow). **(b)** Mark the entry point with the sheathed needle. **(c)** Palpating the anterior acromion to show the direction the needle will go. **(d)** Showing injection being given.

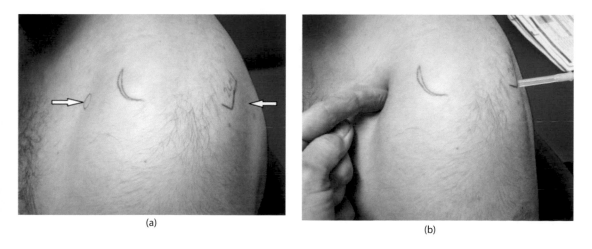

Figure 3.21  Glenohumeral joint injection. **(a)** Showing coracoid at front and injection point at the back (2 cm in and down from posterior corner of acromion). **(b)** Showing direction of injection.

## AC joint

The joint is at an angle of about 70° to the horizontal but can be quite variable. It is a small joint with a volume of about 1 mL. Mark the acromion and the AC joint up and your site of entry (Figure 3.22a through c). Use 1 mL of triamcinolone and 1 mL of 2% lidocaine and put about half in. If you inject and let the pressure off the needle, the fluid should start to come back into the syringe.

In obese people, it can be very difficult to get into the joint; the injection is better done under x-ray control. Warn about paling and thinning of the skin, which can occur with this injection.

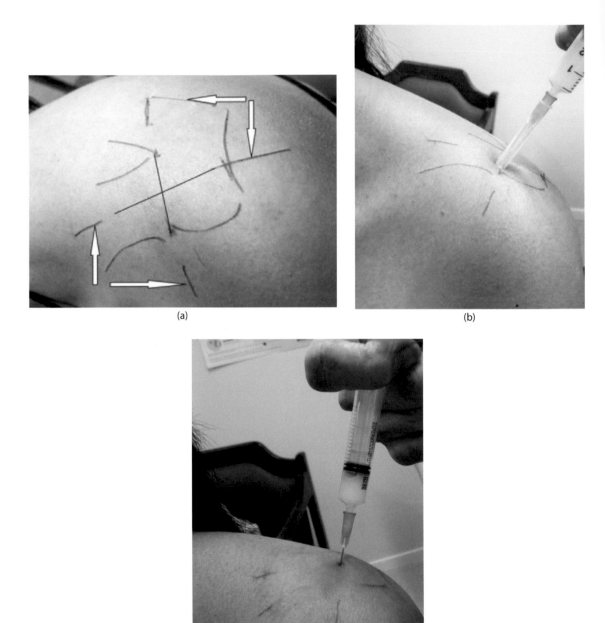

(a)

(b)

(c)

Figure 3.22 Acromioclavicular joint injection. **(a)** Mark surface anatomy then lines which meet at proposed site of injection. Arrows indicate where the lines are which cross at the joint. **(b)** Showing where injection will go. Note angle to vertical. **(c)** Injection being given.

## SUMMARY

- The shoulder joint is really two proper joints (glenohumeral and AC) and two pseudo-joints (subacromial space and scapulothoracic space).
- Shoulder problems are either pain or dislocations (with or without pain).
- Shoulder pain lasting more than 3 weeks is unlikely to settle on its own.
- Shoulders that are painful fall into one of four groups: something nasty (malignancy/infection), the neck, not moving (glenohumeral OA, frozen shoulder, locked posterior dislocation) or normal movement that is painful (impingement +/− cuff disorders and AC joint pain, scapular problems).
- To separate painful shoulders out:
  - Moving the neck creates the 'shoulder pain' = likely the neck
- Will not move it at all = think 'nasty'
- Normal external rotation (compare to the other side) = impingement etc.
- Reduced external rotation (compared to other side) = OA glenohumeral joint/frozen shoulder/locked posterior dislocation
- Remember the red flags (5) and refer: infection, malignancy, fracture, unreduced dislocation, acute cuff tear secondary to trauma.
- Judicious use of steroid injections can be useful. Taking a course to gain information, tips and confidence is useful. Repeated steroid injections with short effect should be avoided.

## Reference

1. Kulkarni R, Gibson J, Brownson P, Thomas M, Rangan A, Carr, AJ, Rees JL. BESS/BOA patient care pathways sub acromial shoulder pain. *Shoulder Elbow*. 2015;7(2):135–143.

# Elbow disorders

KEVIN BOYD

## Introduction

Twenty percent of the population consult their general practitioner (GP) each year with a musculoskeletal condition; 3% of these relate to the elbow.[1] Elbow problems typically present with pain following injury or after repetitive use. Stiffness is often tolerated well and sometimes not recognised in slowly evolving degenerative conditions such as osteoarthritis. Patients with rheumatoid arthritis can have significant symptoms from their elbows with pain, swelling and weakness. Upper limb joints can be protected to a degree in day-to-day activities in ways that the major lower joints cannot. Manual workers and athletes tend to present with problems earlier as their symptoms interfere more readily with work and/or leisure pursuits.

## Anatomy

The elbow is a synovial, hinge joint, incorporating the proximal radioulnar joint. Pronation of the forearm involves the radius rotating around the fixed ulnar to allow positioning of the hand. In this respect, both the proximal and the distal radioulnar joints are important in allowing forearm rotation.

The elbow normally has a large range of motion, typically from 0° (extension), and often several degrees of hyperextension, to approximately 140° (flexion). As the arm fully extends, the olecranon is accommodated in the olecranon fossa of the distal humerus and similarly in full flexion, the coronoid process enters the coronoid fossa anteriorly extending this range. These bony articulations confer relative stability of the elbow joint in these positions. In mid-arc positions, however, stability is determined largely by the ulnar and radial collateral ligaments. On the lateral side, the collateral ligament blends with the annular ligament of the proximal radioulnar joint which permits free rotation of the radial head.

The main flexors of the elbow are the brachialis and the biceps muscles. The attachment of the biceps on the radius also obligates supination of the forearm. The triceps muscle is the main extensor of the elbow with its insertion on the olecranon process.

The forearm muscles are the flexors of the wrist and fingers with their common origin from the medial epicondyle, the extensor group from the lateral epicondyle, and the lateral group (or 'mobile wad') from the lateral supracondylar ridge of the distal humerus. Forearm pronation is mainly provided by pronator teres of the flexor group. The extensor group typically acts as stabilisers of the wrist. The muscle groups also provide dynamic stability control around the elbow joint.

At the level of the elbow, the median nerve is located deeply anteromedially near the brachial artery. The radial nerve, having run down the spiral groove, passes anterolaterally around the elbow. The ulnar nerve passes behind the medial epicondyle in the cubital tunnel (the 'funny bone' area) before entering the forearm flexor muscles. The brachial artery can be palpated medial to the biceps tendon.

## History

Acute injuries typically follow falls onto an outstretched hand, resulting in an indirect force applied to the elbow, causing fracture and/or dislocation. Certain conditions can worsen following injury, for example, early osteoarthritis or tendinopathy. Normal tendons can fail following applied supranormal forces; older degenerative tendons can fail under physiological loads. A history of previous injuries, often as a child, may be important as these injuries can result in residual deformity or acquired deformity through growth disturbance.

Overuse syndromes with an insidious onset are common. Work and leisure activities are important potential causes of repetitive injury. For manual workers, athletes and musicians, both hands are often used equally rather than just the 'dominant' side. Elbow pain may emanate from the joint itself, the adjacent soft tissues (muscles, tendons and nerves) or radiate from elsewhere. Pain can be considered to be medial, lateral, anterior and posterior. Mechanical pain is related to and exacerbated by activity. Tendinopathies typically have stiffness initially followed by a warm-up period and further pain after activity. Provocative and relieving factors should be sought. Night pain may be reflective of a more serious pathology and red flag symptoms should be identified.

Pain and neurological symptoms potentially may radiate from the neck. A C6 radiculopathy produces lateral elbow pain that may be mistaken for the more common lateral elbow tendinopathy (tennis elbow). Some neck pain and stiffness might be expected along with neurological symptoms of numbness, tingling and weakness in the arm.

Bilateral arm symptoms may suggest a central neck cause.

Locking or mechanical jamming symptoms can be seen in degenerative conditions associated with intra-articular loose bodies. Clicking around the elbow is quite an unusual symptom but may reflect a subluxing ulnar nerve or a snapping triceps tendon when experienced medially. Painful clunking laterally, particularly when the arm is loaded through the hand, may be a sign of elbow subluxation or posterolateral instability.

Stiffness is common in osteoarthritis and may be the only clinical feature. Loss of range of motion is often tolerated well and patients may not notice quite significant restriction for some time. Elbow effusions are subtle and patients may complain of 'stiffness' or 'tightness'. Focal swellings may reflect an olecranon bursitis, rheumatoid nodules or gouty tophi. These are usually not painful unless infected or injured.

Nerve problems at the elbow may manifest as symptoms in the hand, most commonly the ulnar nerve (cubital tunnel syndrome). Weakness of the hand or forearm muscles may be a reflection of nerve injury or pain inhibition.

Work-related upper limb disorder (WRULD), previously known as repetitive strain injury, is a complex combination of pain, stiffness, cramp and tingling associated with repetitive movements. This may affect the elbow as part of a more nonspecific upper limb disorder. Diagnosis is usually by exclusion. Treatment is with activity modification and symptom management.

Overhead and throwing athletes are often acutely aware of minor deficits such as loss of throwing or serving speed. Power for these activities are generated through the large muscles of the legs and the back and are then transferred along the 'kinetic chain' via the elbow ultimately to the hand, ball or racquet. The elbow adds little additional power but is vulnerable to biomechanical strains in the mid-range positions where the ligaments are important. Paediatric and adolescent athletes are prone to overuse injuries with their immature skeletons and relative susceptibility to bone (rather than ligament) injury. An expert in treating sporting injuries is often best placed to work with athletes and their coaches in identifying causation of the problem which may involve technical errors or second injuries elsewhere.

## Examination

Examination begins with inspection, though this may be unremarkable. Look for localised or generalised swelling. Bruising usually infers a recent tendon or ligament injury. Isolated swellings posteriorly may reflect olecranon bursitis, gouty tophi or rheumatoid nodules. Rarely skin changes may occur, either in colour or with stiff, shiny tissues, and these might suggest autoimmune, chronic regional pain syndromes or vascular occlusions. Effusions in the elbow joint are often subtle and may be difficult to identify. They are best seen with the elbow flexed, losing the skin dimple just posterior to the radiocapitellar joint. This may reflect a reactive or inflammatory intra-articular process. Intra-articular infections present with a relatively short history, systemic upset and marked painful splinting of the joint.

Assess the carrying angles from the front with elbows extended alongside the body. Asymmetry may suggest an old childhood injury. This is harder to appreciate with a fixed flexion deformity. Range of movement, both flexion/extension and pronation/supination, should be documented accurately. Range does vary between individuals and should be compared to the opposite side. Differences with time can reflect disease progression or indeed resolution. The arms should always go fully straight (0°) but hyperextension of −10° is seen in those with relative flexibility. Similarly, flexion can range from 130° to 150°. A good screening test is to view elbow movements from in front with the arms abducted at 90° to the sides. Differences are easily appreciated in this position. The arms are then brought into the sides to check forearm rotation. A range of 180° would be expected.

Palpation for tenderness should identify all the bony landmarks and tendon attachments. These include the medial and lateral epicondyles and the olecranon process. These bony landmarks should always form an equilateral triangle. The radial head is best defined by passive forearm rotation, feeling its movement beneath the skin. Subluxation of the ulnar nerve happens moving into full flexion. A finger rested on the medial epicondyle while passively flexing the elbow will feel the nerve come up and flick over the epicondyle if unstable. Rarely a 'snapping triceps' tendon (an anatomical variant) may be a cause of similar symptoms and signs.

Mechanical symptoms, if causing enough problem, might justify a surgical opinion.

The territory of any neurological disturbance should be confirmed. These can be dermatomal or related to individual peripheral nerves. Using a central area of each nerve territory provides a good screening tool. These are the pulp of the index finger for the median nerve, the lateral border of the little finger for the ulnar nerve and the first dorsal web space for the radial nerve. Similarly, in terms of power, resisted thumb abduction (median), resisted finger abduction (ulnar) and resisted finger extension (radial) are the best single tests for respective nerve power. Tinel's test may suggest increased local irritability over the cubital tunnel. Peripheral pulses should be assessed. Colour changes, delayed capillary return, nail bed changes and atrophy of the fingertips may be seen in vasculitic processes.

The shoulder and neck should be checked for pain and restriction in motion as radiating symptoms into the arm are not uncommon.

## Special tests

Specific tests may be indicated depending on the suspicions raised by the history and initial examination.

Lateral elbow tendinopathy (tennis elbow) can be suggested by resisted finger or wrist extension leading to localised pain at the lateral epicondyle (Cozen's test). Similarly, resisted pronation for medial elbow tendinopathy (golfer's elbow) will produce medial epicondyle pain. Passive stretch tests can also suggest tendinopathies. For lateral elbow tendinopathy pain, the extensor muscles are passively stretched by pronating the forearm, flexing the wrist and then extending the elbow. For medial elbow tendinopathy, the forearm is supinated, the wrist extended, before extending the elbow fully. These positions can be used by patients to undertake their own stretches.

Valgus and varus stress tests are used for assessment of the medial and lateral collateral ligaments, respectively. Tests are performed in 30° flexion to unlock the olecranon process from the olecranon fossa. As the arm can rotate at the shoulder and give a false impression of movement, the shoulder is placed in full external rotation when assessing the medial structures and in full internal rotation when assessing the lateral structures.

Posterolateral rotatory instability of the elbow is an unusual condition usually seen after a significant fall leading to an injury short of a full dislocation. It is best demonstrated by the 'table top' test. With the patient standing, the hands are fully supinated and then a push up is done on the edge of the table top. A lateral-sided, painful clunk is positive.

A distal biceps tendon rupture is suggested by the 'hook' sign. With the elbow tensed in mid-flexion and supination, it should be possible to hook an index finger around the biceps tendon from the lateral side. Inability to feel a defined tendon suggests a rupture. A 'popeye' sign (bunching of the biceps muscle belly with resistance) can be seen with a distal rupture as well as the more common rupture of long head of biceps proximally.

## Investigations

X-rays should be performed if there is suggestion of a fracture or dislocation. A low threshold for x-ray should be considered in children who have a higher likelihood of fracture compared with adults. X-rays will show osteoarthritic change with joint space narrowing, sclerosis and osteophyte formation and occasionally loose bodies. Early osteoarthritis can be made clinically without the need for imaging. Multiple loose body formation as a consequence of synovial chondromatosis is obvious on x-rays. In children, subtle fractures may present difficulties in interpretation of x-rays because of the multiple ossification centres around the elbow.

Ultrasound is widely available and is the investigation of choice for tendon-related problems. Again tendinopathies are often apparent clinically. Ultrasound will show loss of the normal tendon fibrillar pattern and any neovascularity and identify any tears. Magnetic resonance imaging (MRI) scans show a wide range of soft tissue and bony problems including areas of oedema suggesting injury or bone stress. Subtle osteophytes, loose bodies and other bony abnormalities are best shown by a computed tomography (CT) scan, but typically this would be reserved for secondary care.

Nerve conduction studies are important for assessing ulnar nerve function and the location of any focal nerve compression. As this can occur both proximally and at the level of the wrist, these are usually performed before consideration of surgical ulnar nerve decompression.

## Elbow trauma

The elbow is the second most common joint to dislocate (after the shoulder). Ninety percent of *elbow dislocations* are posterior in direction and usually follow a fall onto an outstretched hand, often affecting children. Acute symptoms of pain, swelling and deformity should lead to an immediate x-ray. Typically, loss of the 'triangle' between the epicondyles and the olecranon process is noticed. Closed reduction is usually achievable with pain relief, sedation and/or a general anaesthetic. The elbow is typically supported in a back slab for 3 weeks to allow the soft tissue injury to settle.

Similar symptoms may reflect a *supracondylar fracture* of the distal humerus. These can be associated with vascular or nerve damage. Assessment of distal pulses, capillary return and nerve function, particularly the ability to perform an 'OK' sign, is essential. Frequently, manipulation with or without percutaneous k-wire fixation is required to stabilise these fractures, and an early orthopaedic opinion is required as surgery becomes technically more difficult with swelling.

Depending on the forces, the radial head or neck may be fractured. An acute effusion is often a sign of haemarthrosis. Subtle intra-articular fractures may be suspected by displacement of the fat pads that normally lie in the olecranon and coronoid fossae by the haemarthrosis creating a 'sail' sign on the lateral elbow x-ray. Palpation of the radial head by passively rotating the forearm while applying pressure along the length of the forearm will highlight any local bony tenderness.

The subcutaneous border of the ulnar is palpable along its length making it readily accessible for identification of *olecranon fractures*. Given the single functioning unit of the forearm, it is unusual to fracture one forearm bone without a second fracture or a dislocation. Consequently, a *Monteggia-type injury* (a proximal ulnar fracture with a dislocated radial head) and a *Galeazzi-type injury* (fracture of the distal radius with dislocation of the ulnar head) can be seen.

Significant elbow fractures and injuries can result in chronic stiffness as a result of scarring. Sometimes heterotopic calcification can occur. If modest and asymptomatic then this can be recognised and left alone.

Tendon ruptures may be partial or complete and include distal biceps insertion or the triceps.

Assessing strength through resisted action and palpation of the contracting tendon is appropriate.

A *pulled elbow* is often seen in preschool children and is felt to reflect a subluxation of the radial head from the annular ligament, typically caused by a pull along an extended arm. The ensuing pain is often hard to qualify. An attempt to 'reduce' the radial head with longitudinal pressure along the forearm while rotating the hand can result in a reduction clunk, but this is often unsatisfying. Reassurance and a sling for a couple of days will usually result in spontaneous resolution.

Whereas bony injuries are more common following falls in children, the possibility of *non-accidental injury (NAI)* should always be borne in mind. Multiple attendances at the emergency department, inconsistent stories, injuries of differing age and abnormal child/carer interactions may all be suggestive of NAI. Remember, children who are not yet walking cannot fall over on their own.

## Chronic elbow pain

Chronic or overuse elbow pain can be approached based on anatomical structures, considering lateral, medial, anterior and posterior areas.

## Lateral elbow pain

*Lateral elbow tendinopathy* provides a better description for the term *tennis elbow*, though this is widely understood by patients and clinicians alike. Epicondylitis is misleading when the pathology is a degenerative tendon process. The worst pain is felt over the conjoint tendon insertion on to the anterior aspect of the lateral epicondyle rather than the lateral bony prominence itself. The causation of tendinopathy is multifactorial though the final pathway is biomechanical overload and microscopic failure. Tendon quality deteriorates with age and genetic factors are important in some individuals.

Lateral elbow tendinopathy is common with an estimated prevalence of 1%–3%.[2] Men and women are equally affected, most commonly in the fifth and sixth decades of life. Populations that involve lifting, carrying and repetitive mechanical activities are more likely to develop and have limitations from this problem.

Those with mild day to day symptoms often self-manage. First-line treatments in primary care should include prolonged stretches (at least 30 seconds, similar to those used in diagnosis – see 'Special tests' above) and strengthening exercises to help recondition the tendons. The tendons have failed under loading but do respond to mechanical stimuli and therefore with training can readapt. Numerous exercise programmes have been proposed though evidence seems to suggest an eccentric strengthening programme (i.e. muscles working while lengthening) is most effective. Improvements are not seen immediately and given the relatively low-metabolic nature of tendons, change is seen over months rather than weeks. A physiotherapist can advise on such a programme although home exercises programmes involving loading with water bottles, walking sticks or hammers are readily available. There is little evidence to support the use of electrophysical modalities such as therapeutic ultrasound, diathermy or acupuncture though there are few adverse features either. Additional self-help with firm local massage and the use of a counterforce brace or clasp applied over the muscle belly of the extensor muscle group are of benefit in some patients.

Injections of a long-acting steroid and local anaesthetic have traditionally been offered for tendinopathies. Modern understanding suggests the benefit of this may be at best short lived and can cause the condition to worsen in the longer term. If a patient can manage without an injection then this may best be avoided, at least initially, whilst physiotherapy is undertaken. If the level of pain indicates an injection is required, then this remains an acceptable practice. Patients should be counselled regarding side effects and the injection is given into the conjoint tendon anterior to the lateral epicondyle. Most patients with lateral elbow tendinopathy will receive a period of useful improvement following a steroid injection. The diagnosis may need reconsideration if this is not the case.

New methods of treatment have attracted attention such as injections with whole autologous blood (ABI), platelet rich plasma (PRP) or extracorporeal shockwave therapy (EWST). There is some evidence to support the use of these and while some patients experience useful benefit, the place and cost-effectiveness of these remain unclear. The National Institute for Health and Clinical Excellence (NICE) has issued guidance[3,4] suggesting that the techniques are safe but need close audit and further research before general recommendation can be made. Which technique is more beneficial in which patient remains unclear, though these techniques may be offered in specialist departments.

Surgical intervention remains an option for patients who have failed a comprehensive programme of non-operative measures. Surgery most commonly involves an open debridement of the grossly abnormal tendon leading to benefit in 80%–90% of patients. This is normally performed as a day case under a full anaesthetic and is typically tolerated well. Strengthening exercises remain an important part of postoperative rehabilitation.

Rarely, *entrapment of the posterior interosseous nerve* can lead to lateral elbow pain. Typically, this is more distal to the common extensor origin over the extensor muscles. Often some subtle neurological symptoms are found here and provocative tests for lateral elbow tendinopathy are absent. Nerve condition studies can confirm the diagnosis.

*Posterolateral rotatory instability* leads to laterally based elbow discomfort and mechanical symptoms. Typically, these are provoked by particular indirect loading activities, and surgical reconstruction is often required.

*Congenital dislocation of the radial head* can occur either as isolated problems or as part of a wider syndrome, e.g., Klinefelter's syndrome or Ehlers–Danlos syndrome. This is often tolerated well in the first two decades and treatment is usually symptomatic. Radial head excision can be considered in skeletally mature patients with focal degenerative change.

*Referred pain* is more likely on the lateral side of the elbow and proximal sources of pain in the shoulder and neck should be considered.

## Medial elbow pain

*Medial elbow tendinopathy (golfer's elbow)* has many features in keeping with lateral elbow tendinopathy, though it is 10 times less common. Clearly, the location of pain and the provocative tests differ but non-operative and surgical management options have similar indications and results (see above). Any active intervention needs careful consideration of the ulnar nerve that is located behind the medial epicondyle.

*Ulnar nerve neuropathy* can lead to pain and hypersensitivity over the inner elbow. Paraesthesia is typically felt over the ulnar one and half digits,

often with altered sensation. There may be wasting and weakness of ulnar nerve innervated muscles in the hand. Nerve condition studies can confirm localised slowing of nerve function at the level of the elbow. Surgery is indicated for troublesome symptoms but inevitably can only address compressive lesions. Paraesthesiae are most reliably addressed by surgery, but long-standing weakness is unlikely to recover fully. Surgery involves decompression of nerve as it runs through the cubital tunnel with or without an anterior transposition of the nerve. Mechanical clicking over the medial side often with radiating neurological symptoms may reflect a subluxing ulnar nerve in which case an anterior transposition should be performed. A snapping triceps accessory tendon may be an unusual cause of mechanical symptoms in this area.

Acute sprains of the medial collateral ligament or strains of the common flexor muscles can occur through falls or throwing mechanisms of injury. Repetitive throwing can lead to chronic stretch of the medial collateral ligament injuries with repeated valgus strains, the *valgus extension overload syndrome (VEOLS)*. This can also lead to posteromedial impingement of the olecranon within the olecranon fossa as it snaps into full extension. Surgery to augment the stretched ligament with or without removal of osteophytes may be indicated.

## Anterior elbow pain

Pain associated with **osteoarthritis** may be poorly defined (and can be felt mainly posteriorly). It is often felt deep within the elbow but fortunately may be relatively minor even with quite advanced disease. It can present with localised disease, for example, in the radiocapitellar joint laterally. Pain is provoked by movements into end range and when carrying weights. Initial treatment is symptomatic with maintenance of active movements, analgesia and physiotherapy. Steroid injections can be considered for short-term relief. Significant loss of functional range and/or loose body formation can be addressed by surgical debridement using arthroscopic or open approaches. Improvements in pain and in range of motion can be anticipated, but normality is never achieved.

Inflammatory arthropathies affect the elbow though rarely as the first joint to present. *Rheumatoid arthritis* has both juvenile and adult forms leading to pain and stiffness and, in late cases, instability. Aggressive early management with disease modifying agents is indicated and surgical salvage is now less common. Total elbow replacement is more successful in rheumatoid disease, compared with osteoarthritis, as the demands placed on the elbow are less.

Rarely in teenage patients, *osteochondritis* dissecans can affect the elbow as a cause of pain, restricted movements and/or loose body formation. X-rays and 3D imaging may be required to make a firm diagnosis. Treatment is usually symptomatic. Similarly, in juvenile patients (aged 5–12 years), a spontaneous osteochondrosis of the capitellum (*Panner's disease*) can occur. Treatment here is again symptomatic. It should be borne in mind that child athletes can present with overuse stress injuries affecting the bones and the epiphyseal or apophyseal growth plates around the elbow. Repetitive loading from throwing or weight-bearing activities, such as arm stands in gymnastics, are often responsible and close co-operation with the coach and parents is required to manage such problems.

The biceps tendon is an obvious anterior structure at the elbow. Overuse activities with localising pain on palpation of the tendon or on resistance may reflect *biceps tendinopathy*. Analgesia, modification of activity and progressive retraining of the tendon with physiotherapy may be required. *Biceps rupture* should be considered with any acute onset associated with bruising, swelling and a potential change in shape in the contracted muscle belly. Early surgery (within a few weeks) is easier but non-operative management with acceptance of a modest loss of strength (~20%) may be preferred.

## Posterior elbow pain

The triceps tendon is the main posterior structure at the elbow. *Triceps tendinopathy* occurs usually due to weight training activities. Pain is localised to the tendon on passive stretching and active resistance. The integrity should be confirmed clinically, or with imaging if necessary. Again modification of activity, symptomatic management and physiotherapy will be helpful.

*Olecranon bursitis* is quite common after recurrent irritation or repeated pressure resting on the elbow (*student's elbow*). The lesions are soft and cystic and will transilluminate. Aspiration leads to clear, mildly viscous fluid but frequently, the collection reoccurs. Instillation of steroid has not been shown to make recurrence any less likely. They are tolerated well but may be a cosmetic concern if large. Redness and pain may reflect a secondary infection that requires active management with antibiotics, aspiration or surgical drainage. Other solid posterior elbow lesions such as gouty tophi or rheumatoid nodules may occasionally require surgical excision due to nuisance or cosmetic reasons. Optimisation of medical management may help control their development.

---

### SUMMARY

In children, elbow trauma, such as fractures and dislocations, is quite common. X-rays, interpreted by an experienced clinician, should be obtained if suspected. Adult patients tend to experience degenerative conditions such as tendinopathies and osteoarthritis. Many can be diagnosed by clinical assessment and managed with simple measures and advice in general practice. Secondary care can be consulted after failure of first-line treatments.

How to inject for lateral elbow tendinopathy (tennis elbow):

- Make the patient sit or lie with elbow flexed at 90°.
- Draw up to 1 mL 1% lidocaine and 40 mg (1 mL) triamcinolone.
- Change to a fresh 23G needle.
- Identify landmarks and cleanse the skin.
- Inject the tendon 'peppering' 0.2 mL aliquots in the 1 cm$^3$ area anterior to the lateral epicondyle.

## Resources

1. http://www.nhs.uk/Conditions/Tennis-elbow/Pages/Treatment.aspx
2. http://www.nhs.uk/Conditions/Tendonitis/Pages/Introduction.aspx
3. http://www.csp.org.uk/your-health/exercise-advice-all-ages-fitness/exercise-advice-videos
4. http://cks.nice.org.uk/tennis-elbow#!scenario
5. http://cks.nice.org.uk/olecranon-bursitis#!scenario
6. http://www.arthritisresearchuk.org/arthritis-information/conditions/elbow-pain.aspx

# References

1. Royal College of General Practitioners – Birmingham Research Unit. Annual prevalence report. 2006.
2. Bisset L, Coombes B, Vicenzino B. Tennis elbow. *BMJ Clin Evid*. June 2011, http://clinicalevidence.bmj.com/x/systematic-review/1117/overview.html
3. NICE. Autologous blood injection for tendinopathy. NICE interventional procedure guidance [IPG438]. January 2013, https://www.nice.org.uk/guidance/ipg438
4. NICE. Extracorporeal shockwave therapy for refractory tennis elbow. NICE interventional procedure guidance [IPG313]. August 2009, https://www.nice.org.uk/guidance/ipg313

# 5

# Hand and wrist disorders

BIJAYENDRA SINGH

The hand and wrist consist of 29 bones, 29 joints and 29 tendons and muscles. They are connected by a multiple ligaments providing a delicate balance to provide optimum function. Their function is integral to every act of daily living in the young and old. They are the most active part of body. Problems of the wrist and hand can be due to trauma, overuse or general wear and tear. They are one of the most commonly searched and published areas of research in the scientific world. The hand and wrist are the least protected joints and extremely vulnerable to injury. The history can be vague and difficult. Hence, it's important to focus on the answers and examine the relevant parts and conduct appropriate investigations.

Important factors to consider include age, occupation, handedness and the main complaints. It's also important to know any activities that exacerbate or relive the symptoms. A history of previous injury or surgery is also important.

The hand and wrist are common sites for arthritis and trauma. Other inflammatory conditions like rheumatoid arthritis can also affect the hand and its function. The fingers can become deformed and can cause pressure on nerves in the hand.

Surgery comes in various forms to reconstruct tendons/ligaments or remove diseased and inflamed parts.

## What is carpal tunnel syndrome?

Carpal tunnel syndrome (CTS) is the most common entrapment neuropathy in the body. This is due to the median nerve getting trapped/compressed as it passes under the transverse carpal ligament (TCL) at the wrist (carpal – from the Greek word karpos, meaning 'wrist') (Figure 5.1a). This can be dynamic or static.

## What is carpal tunnel?

The carpus (wrist) is formed by the eight bones on the dorsal side and is covered by the TCL on the volar aspect. The TCL attaches to the tuberosity of the scaphoid and trapezium laterally to the hamate and pisiform on the medial side. Palmaris longus passes volar to the rest of tendons and merges with the flexor retinaculum to become continuous with the palmar fascia. The contents of the carpal tunnel are the flexor pollicis, flexor digitorum superficialis and flexor digitorum profundus tendons apart from the median nerve.

## What is the chance of getting CTS?

The prevalence of CTS varies according to the population. There is wide variation and it is less commonly seen in the Asian and Afro-Caribbean ethnicities. It's generally accepted that between 3% and 6% of population have CTS. It's more common in females by about 5–10 times as compared to males and also increases with age.

## What causes CTS?

It is widely believed that there is raised pressure in the carpal tunnel due to a variety of reasons thus giving rise to the term 'entrapment' neuropathy. The increased pressure in the tunnel may have an obvious cause, but in most cases, these are not present and such cases are termed 'idiopathic' CTS.

The secondary causes and associations are varied but the common ones are as follows:

- Pregnancy
- Rheumatoid arthritis
- Trauma – following distal radius fracture
- Hypothyroid (especially newly diagnosed)
- Diabetes
- Obesity
- Abnormal tissue in the carpal tunnel

## How do you diagnose CTS?

## Symptoms

The diagnosis is mainly clinical based on the patient's symptoms and signs. The typical symptoms are tingling and numbness in the radial two-thirds of the hand, and electric shock-like sensations in the fingers. Occasionally, patients get pain radiating

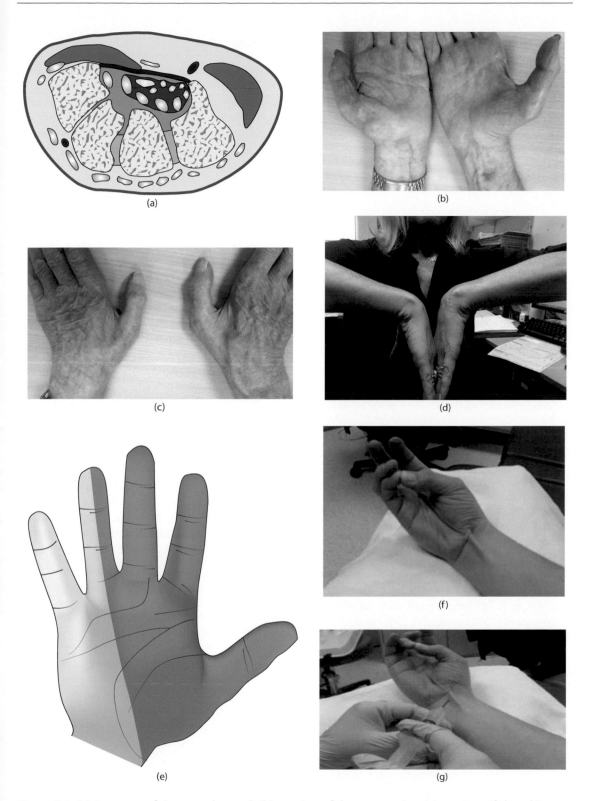

Figure 5.1 **(a)** Anatomy of the carpal tunnel; **(b)** wasting of thenar muscles; **(c)** wasting of dorsal inter-ossei; **(d)** Phalen's test; **(e)** sensory distribution of median nerve; **(f)** identification of palmaris longus; **(g)** steroid injection for CTS.

up from the wrist to the forearm and elbow (anti-dromic). Symptoms are made worse by using a keyboard, holding a phone and driving. Patients often wake up at night with pins and needles and will typically describe that they have to hang the hand at edge of bed or shake it away. Always ask for symptoms of involvement more proximally especially cervical spine involvement. Check if the patient has any radicular symptoms down the arm.

## Signs

On inspection, look for any wasting of muscles of the thenar eminence (Figure 5.1b and c) which usually suggests severe CTS and may be beyond recovery. Phalen's test involves flexing the wrist as much as possible and will elicit the patient's symptoms (Figure 5.1d). Tinel's sign is demonstrated by tapping on the wrist crease to elicit recurrence of pins and needles or a shooting sensation in the fingers to assess irritability of the nerve. Test the sensation of the hand – the median nerve supplies the radial three and half digits (Figure 5.1e). If there is numbness, this again is a poor prognostic factor as the sensation does not improve predictably, and the patient should be warned about this. Always check for any evidence for a higher lesion.

## Are there any special investigations to diagnose CTS?

Electromyographic (EMG) or nerve conduction studies (NCS) are the diagnostic tests to confirm CTS. Unfortunately, not all patients with classical symptoms of CTS have a positive test, but it certainly helps in counselling patients about the outcome as it has been shown that patients with symptoms of CTS but negative EMG studies have a slightly less predictable outcome.

Plain radiographs are indicated if the patient has restricted wrist movements leading to pain to rule out any underlying arthritis, or the symptoms are atypical.

## How do you treat CTS?

The mainstay of CTS is surgical decompression, but in the early stages or with mild symptoms, non-surgical treatment may be tried. Non-surgical treatment is especially useful if there is a secondary/temporary cause of CTS, i.e. third trimester of pregnancy.

## Non-surgical

**Bracing or splinting:** The median nerve is compressed when the wrist is flexed. A simple off-the-shelf splint that can be bought from chemist shop keeps the wrist in slightly extended position and helps with the symptoms of CTS. This is especially helpful for night-time symptoms or certain daytime activities like driving, answering phone calls etc., which precipitate the symptoms.

**Medications:** Simple medications like non-steroidal anti-inflammatory drugs (NSAIDs), such as diclofenac or ibuprofen, may help relieve some symptoms. Oral steroids have been tried, but the results are not convincing.

**Activity changes:** Activity modifications or workplace adjustments can help relieve some symptoms of CTS.

**Steroid injections:** A corticosteroid injection frequently used often provides relief, but symptoms may come back. This is done next to the carpal tunnel – easily identified by asking to pinch the thumb to ring finger to make the palmaris longus taut. The needle is inserted just next to the palmaris longus (Figure 5.1f and g).

## Surgical treatment

The decision to proceed to surgery usually depends on the severity of symptoms and if non-surgical management has failed to relieve the symptoms. In cases where the symptoms interfere with patient's activities of daily living (ADL) or with muscle wasting or numbness, surgery is recommended as the first step.

## What are the outcomes and complications after CTS surgery?

Good to excellent results are seen in over 90% of cases. Some patients may have pillar pain or scar tenderness for a few weeks after surgery. If the patient already has muscle wasting and numbness, the recovery is slightly less predictable.

## What is ganglion?

Ganglion is the most common cause of a lump on the wrist. This commonly arises from the joint itself when a small rent in the joint lining (synovium) forms a little pouch. This gradually becomes bigger and lies in between the tendons. It can also arise out of tendon sheaths or ligaments (Figure 5.2a).

## What are the causes of ganglion?

The exact reason is unknown. It is most commonly seen in younger age group patients – certainly aged less than 45 years. It is more common in women than in men. It can be seen more frequently in people doing gymnastic or repeated loading/stress of wrists. If an older patient presents with ganglion cyst it is often related to arthritis in the wrist joint.

## What problems do patients get because of ganglion?

In the early stages when the ganglion is forming, patients will present with ache in the wrist usually after activity. When the ganglion has formed, it will be a visible lump – most commonly on the dorsum of the wrist. If the ganglion gets bigger, then it can cause local pressure symptoms and can restrict movements (Figure 5.2b), but a smaller ganglion is often obscure and may be hidden under the tendons and fascia. Most of the dorsal ganglions produce no other symptoms. However, if it's on the volar side then it may cause pressure on the nerves and vessels that pass across the joint leading to tingling, numbness, pain and, in rare and severe cases, muscle wasting. Large cysts, even if not painful, can cause local mechanical symptoms and/or cosmetic concern. The majority of cysts around the nail are due to underlying osteoarthritis and it's important to look for symptoms related to OA.

## How do you treat ganglion?

The majority of patients with ganglion can be treated non-operatively with reassurance and observation. Fifty percent of these lumps disappear with time, about 30% stay the same and 20% may get a bit bigger over a period of 3–5 years. You will hardly see a patient who presents with a 3–5-year history of lump. Remember to treat the cause of the underlying ganglion.

## Non-surgical treatment

- **Observation:** The natural history of ganglion suggests that early surgery is not recommended and hence keeping an eye on the lump at the initial consultation is appropriate.
- **Aspiration:** If the ganglion is large and the patient is not keen on surgical excision, then the ganglion can be aspirated. To do this, the area is numbed with local anaesthetic, and the cyst is punctured with a needle multiple times in an attempt to aspirate the fluid (or often the fluid is dispersed in soft tissue). Some surgeons infiltrate hyaluronic acid after aspiration – this has not shown to be any superior than simple aspiration. Usually following aspiration, the cyst returns.

## Surgical treatment

Surgery involves removal of the ganglion. This can be done in the open or arthroscopically and will entail leaving a small opening in the wrist capsule (capsulotomy). The main complication following this is recurrence in about 10%–15%.

## What is trigger finger?

Trigger finger/thumb causes clicking and locking of the involved digit. There is usually an underlying

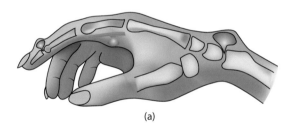

(a)

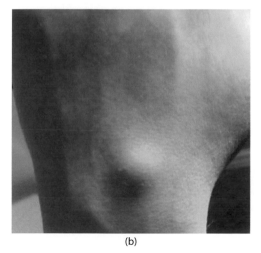

(b)

Figure 5.2 **(a)** Common sites of ganglion cysts; **(b)** dorsal wrist ganglion.

tenosynovitis of tendon sheath which causes it to thicken. Sometimes, it may be permanently locked down.

## What happens in trigger finger?

The flexor tendon synovium can become inflamed and thickened for a variety of reasons. As the tendon passes across the mouth of A1 pulley, it starts to jam and causes bunching of the synovium. This then thickens and forms a nodule, which can get stuck at the opening of the A1 pulley. The patient may feel a clicking sensation or jamming of the finger as the tendon slips through the tight area, and the finger can be straightened with shooting pain (Figure 5.3).

## What causes trigger finger?

The exact cause for trigger finger is usually unknown. There are some factors that may predispose certain individuals to get triggering in the fingers:

- More common in women than men.
- Occurs commonly between the ages of 30 and 60 years.
- Patients with diabetes and inflammatory arthritis, i.e. rheumatoid arthritis have a higher risk.

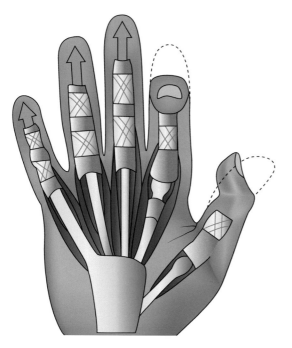

Figure 5.3 Location of A1 pulley causing triggering.

## How do you diagnose trigger finger?

Usually the history clinches the diagnosis. On examining the patient, one may find a tender lump/nodule in the palm at the flexion crease of the fingers – the mouth of the A1 pulley. There may be some swelling around the mouth of the A1 pulley of the finger. On moving the finger, it may be possible to elicit the locking or often just a clicking sensation as trying to lock the finger may be too painful.

## What is the treatment for trigger finger?

The mainstay of initial treatment is non-surgical in the form of rest and steroid injections.

## Steroid injections

An injection of a corticosteroid – a powerful anti-inflammatory medication – around the opening of tendon sheath helps to alleviate the symptoms, but the relief is unpredictable and variable. If the patient has a long history of triggering, or if there is a hard nodule palpable at the A1 pulley then injections are less likely to be successful but still worth a try (Figure 5.3).

## Surgery

The goal of surgery is to relieve the symptom of clicking and locking. This is done by opening the A1 pulley and freeing the tendon sheath so that the tendon can glide through freely. This is usually done as a day case, most commonly under local anaesthesia. The surgery is performed through a small incision in the palm taking care of the neurovascular bundle, which is close by. The A1 pulley is released and it heals in a lengthened way allowing the tendon to glide easily.

## What are the possible complications of surgery?

Complications following surgery for trigger finger/thumb release are rare but can include the following:

- Damage to the digital nerve and vessels
- Incomplete extension – due to persistent tightness of the tendon sheath

- Persistent triggering – due to incomplete release of the sheath
- Bowstringing – due to excessive release of the sheath
- Infection – rare

## What is de Quervain's disease?

This is tendinosis and tenosynovitis of the tendons affecting the first extensor compartment. This can cause pain and swelling around the thumb (Figure 5.4a).

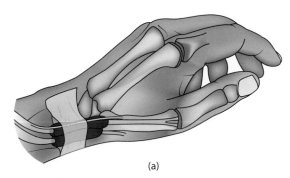

(a)

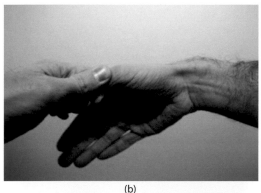

(b)

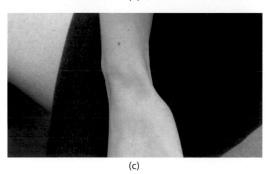

(c)

Figure 5.4 **(a)** First extensor compartment tendons; **(b)** Finkelstein's test; **(c)** skin discoloration after steroid injection.

## Can you explain the anatomy and pathology?

There are six compartments on the dorsum (extensor) of the wrist. The first compartment is where two of the main tendons – the abductor pollicis longus (APL) and extensor pollicis brevis (EPB) to the thumb pass through the extensor retinaculum. The tendons are inflamed and thickened due to a variety of reasons and this results in increased friction and pain with certain thumb and wrist movements.

## What is the cause of de Quervain's disease?

In the majority of cases, the exact cause remains unknown. It is more commonly seen in situations where there may be 'water retention', e.g. last trimester of pregnancy, newly diagnosed rheumatoid (inflammatory) arthritis and post-injury.

## What are the symptoms and signs of de Quervain's disease?

Pain is felt over the thumb and on the lateral side of the wrist. The pain usually occurs gradually but may suddenly appear after minor trauma. The pain can often radiate up the forearm. It's usually made worse when using the thumb for gripping/grasping or twisting movements. Sometimes, there may be swelling around the radial styloid, which can be either soft or hard. Patients may describe a catching or snapping sensation.

Diagnosis is confirmed by Finkelstein's test (Figure 5.4b) which is performed by hyperflexing the thumb, keeping the wrist stable. But do not grab the thumb in the palm as this will cause pain in most people due to irritation of the superficial radial nerve.

## Non-surgical treatment

- **Splints:** If the thumb/wrist is painful then a splint to support the thumb may provide pain relief especially in the third trimester of pregnancy.
- **Anti-inflammatory medication (NSAIDs):** This may help reduce swelling and relieve pain.
- **Avoiding activities that cause pain and swelling:** This may allow the symptoms to go away on their own.
- **Corticosteroid injection:** This is a powerful anti-inflammatory medication and injection

around the tendon sheath will reduce swelling and pain and is useful in secondary cases, i.e. third trimester of pregnancy.

## Surgical treatment

Surgery is recommended if symptoms persist after non-surgical treatment. This is usually performed under local anaesthesia injected around the painful area on an outpatient basis. A transverse incision is made over the first extensor compartment and the tendons are released – and as they heal, it allows more space for the tendon to glide. One must carefully look for multiple septa in the compartment.

## What are the possible complications of surgery?

One possible complication is inadequate release if the surgeon fails to realise that there is more than one compartment in the tendon. The superficial radial nerve is very close to the tendons and there is a small risk of injury which can cause painful neuroma.

The carpometacarpal joint (CMCJ) of the thumb is a very mobile joint that connects the trapezium and the thumb metacarpal. This allows movements like gripping and pinching. This also means that it is at a high risk of developing osteoarthritis.

Arthritis of the base of the thumb is about 7–8 times more common in women than in men. Epidemiological studies show about one-third of women over the age of 45 years have radiological changes but the vast majority of them are asymptomatic. The common age when this occurs is between 40 and 60 years. A history of previous fracture or other injuries to the joint has shown to increase the risk of developing this condition.

## How do you diagnose CMCJ arthritis?

The patients usually present with pain following activities that involve gripping or pinching, such as turning a key, opening a door or opening jars. They may also have swelling and aching at the base of thumb. They may also have some reduction of strength in gripping or pinching activities. Sometimes, the main complaint is related to the appearance of the thumb.

The history usually clinches the diagnosis. There is squaring of the palm with swelling and tenderness at the CMCJ (Figure 5.5a). In the early

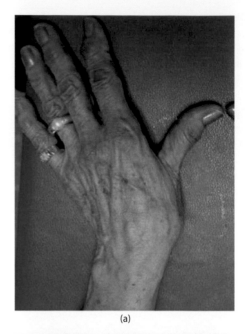
(a)

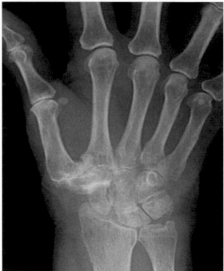
(b)

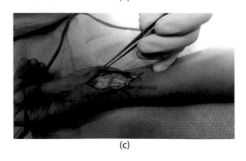
(c)

Figure 5.5 **(a)** Clinical picture of thumb base arthritis; **(b)** typical radiological appearance; **(c)** superficial radial nerve.

stages, a thumb grind test may be undertaken to elicit the symptoms. Plain radiographs will confirm the diagnosis (Figure 5.5b).

## Management

### Non-surgical treatment

In the early stages, the use of NSAIDs, splints and icing may help. A corticosteroid injection done under image guidance provides good relief of pain, but the duration of pain relief is unpredictable. This can be repeated after 3–6 months if required.

### Surgical treatment

There are a variety of options to treat CMCJ arthritis. They can be divided into three groups: fusion, replacement or excision.

**Fusion:** This is usually preferred in the young and manual labourers.

**Replacement:** There are numerous replacement options available designed to maintain the height of the thumb. However, there is no evidence that replacement is superior to any other treatment measure. There is also a higher complication rate following this procedure.

**Excision:** The most common treatment involves excision of the trapezium with or without a ligament suspension arthroplasty. Simple excision of the trapezium has been shown to have equally good results as other surgical options. It's the most reliable option with the fewest complications; the addition of suspension arthroplasty using one of the tendons has been shown to reduce the loss of height.

## What are the possible complications of surgery?

This is usually a very safe surgery, but common complications include damage to the superficial radial nerve (Figure 5.5c) which must be protected throughout the procedure. The other complications include ongoing pain, complex regional pain syndrome (CRPS) and weakness.

Osteoarthritis of the hand is common and generally affects older people.

## What are the symptoms of arthritis of the hand?

The majority of the arthritis affecting the hand is asymptomatic. The symptoms are very variable –

nodular thickening, pain, irritation of local tendon, ligament or nerve, deformity and functional problems. Some joints may become swollen and stiff after use. Some patients develop *ganglion (mucus) cysts* (Figure 5.6) around the distal joint. Most of these joints become 'stable and asymptomatic' over a period of time.

## How do you treat arthritis of the hand?

The treatment depends on the symptoms of the patient. Often explaining the condition and natural history may help the patient deal with the condition. The vast majority of patients initially can be treated non-surgically.

## Non-surgical treatment

This involves activity modification, NSAIDs, splinting and rest. Certain medications like chondroitin sulphate and glucosamine have shown good clinical outcome, but their usefulness has not been proved scientifically. This is available as a food supplement and personally I have seen plenty of patients who have had benefit with this. I would suggest using 1500 mg of glucosamine per day for at least 6 months to notice any difference. Either steroid injections in the joint or intramuscular injections (multiple joint involvement) are often helpful with the pain. If the patient has other symptoms, this may need to be addressed separately.

## Surgical treatment

Surgery is considered if non-surgical treatment fails to improve symptoms, and there is significant

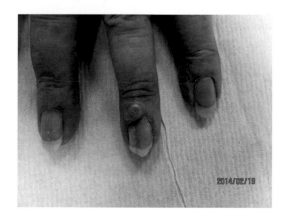

Figure 5.6 Mucus cyst.

pain or disability. The surgical treatment depends on the symptoms and may include excision of cyst, excision of joint, fusion of joint, decompression of nerve or synovectomy.

## What is Dupuytren's contracture?

Dupuytren's contracture (DC) (Figure 5.7a) is a genetic condition that commonly affects the hands and ulnar two digits. It causes one or more of the fingers, on one or both hands, to bend into the palm of the hand. The exact cause is unknown but it is known to run in families and is supposed to be of Viking ancestry.

## Why does DC occur?

The exact cause is unknown, but there are certain risk factors which are as follows:

- Generally, occurs in patients over 60 years of age.
- Men are about 10 times more commonly affected than women.
- Northern European or Scandinavian ancestry.
- It often runs in families (hereditary).
- Associated with excessive alcohol intake.
- Associated with diabetes, seizure medication.

## How do patients with DC present?

The normal tissue in the hand becomes thickened (Figure 5.7b) and presents in one of the following forms:

**Nodules:** The condition starts with formation of nodules in the palm. They may be painful or can cause local irritation especially in patients who handle hard objects.

**Bands of tissue:** The nodules over a period coalesce and form cords in the palm and finger.

**Curled fingers:** Once the cords have 'grown enough', they start to gradually pull the finger towards the palm. This causes difficulty in getting the finger straight, grasping large objects and getting the hands in a pocket.

When you see a patient, especially under the age of 50 years, with suspected DC, always examine or ask about any involvement of the feet or his penis as this may suggest an aggressive disease. He may also have some thickening of tissue on the dorsum of metacarpophalangeal (MCPJ) – *Garrod's pad* (Figure 5.7c), which again suggests aggressive disease.

## When should a patient be referred for an opinion from a hand surgeon?

I would suggest doing a simple test which can be taught to patients. If the patients cannot get their hand flat on a firm surface like a table, or if the palm cups or patients have any functional problems, then they should be referred to a hand surgeon.

## How do you treat DC?

DC is a genetic condition and hence there is no 'cure' as such. The deformity and lumps can be controlled using a variety of techniques. The condition is slowly progressive over a few years and hence a watchful wait can be adopted until it causes functional problems.

## Non-surgical treatment

There is no proven non-surgical treatment which reliably helps patients.

## Surgical treatment

Surgery is recommended when it causes functional problems; patients may have trouble with ADL such as grasping things, washing their face without poking their eyes and getting their hands in pockets (Figure 5.7d).

## Fasciectomy

This is the most common surgery performed for DC. In this, the surgeon will make a zig-zag cut in the hand and remove the diseased tissue. Sometimes, the wound is left open and allowed to heal gradually. Skin grafting may be needed, especially in severe cases and recurrent disorders.

## Needle fasciotomy

The cords in the fingers can be cut using a needle or a small blade. In this technique, the surgeon uses a thick needle (size 18/19 G) and after local anaesthetic cuts the cord in the hand. This is usually reserved for elderly frail patients or those who are anaesthetically not fit for surgery. There is an increased risk of recurrence following this procedure.

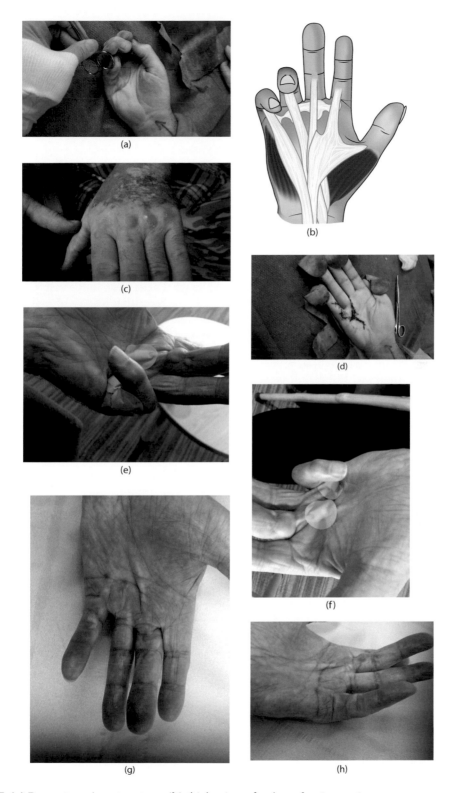

Figure 5.7 **(a)** Dupuytrens' contracture; **(b)** thickening of palmar fascia causing contracture; **(c)** Garrod's pads; **(d)** after fasciectomy; **(e)** Dupuytren's contracture after Xiapex injection; **(f)** Dupuytren's contracture after XIapex injection; **(g and h)** after manipulation following Xiapex.

## What are the newer developments in Dupuytren's disease?

There is an enzyme (Xiapex) injection which breaks down the tough bands by lysis. This has been in use for last 5 years and shown good results and similar recurrence rates to surgery (Figure 5.7e through h).

The technique involves injecting a small amount of enzyme in the cord (disease tissue). This is then followed by a manipulation of the involved finger between 24 and 48 hours under a local anaesthesia. This is done as an outpatient procedure.

## Complications

**Scar:** The scar in the hand and palm will be firm to the touch and tender for 4–6 weeks. This usually settles by massaging the area with moisturising cream once the wound has healed.

**Infection:** This is rare following primary DC surgery. There is a slightly increased risk in revision surgery and when skin grafting has been performed.

**Nerve damage:** Injury to the digital nerves is an uncommon complication following primary surgery. This is seen usually after revision surgery or when the deformity is significant. Sometimes on trying to stretch an extremely bent finger, the nerve may be put on stretch.

**Recurrence:** As DC is a genetic condition, it cannot be cured. The disease can progress, i.e. occur in other hand/fingers, or can reoccur after initial treatment. There is a high recurrence rate after needle fasciotomy – up to as high as 50%. After a fasciectomy, this reduces to 35% and for dermofascietomy it is even lower, around 8%.

**CRPS:** This is uncommon but can have devastating effects. In its mild form, 5% patients have it and it often leads to pain and stiffness in the hands and fingers. In severe cases, the patient may not be able to use the hand for months and may require the input of a pain specialist.

**Degree of correction/recurrence:** This depends primarily on the joint that is involved and secondarily on the amount of deformity. The MCPJ can be fully corrected even with severe deformities, whilst the proximal interphalangeal joint (PIPJ) is resistant to correction even when more than 15°–20°. Hence, the threshold to refer patients should be low if their PIPJ is affected.

**Loss of finger/amputation:** Following primary DC surgery, this is a rare complication. It may result in patients whose fingers have been operated on a number of times. Amputation may be offered as a treatment to an elderly patient with significant deformity who cannot comply with rehabilitation.

## Therapy

This is a very important part of treatment for DC. It's essential to have a good hand therapist to help mobilise and reduce the risk of complications after surgery for DC.

This is commonly a bacterial infection affecting the flexor/extensor tendon sheath in the hand.

## How does tendon sheath infection happen?

Although it's not clear, in the vast majority of cases, there is a preceding history of penetrating injury, often not treated well. In the extensor tendon, it's often due to human bite or punching someone's teeth

## How do you diagnose flexor sheath infection?

Patients with flexor sheath infection (FSI) may present after a penetrating injury, with complaints of pain, redness (Figure 5.8a) and fever. It's important to look for *Kanavel's cardinal signs* of flexor tendon sheath infection, which are as follows:

- Fusiform swelling (Figure 5.8b)
- Tenderness along the flexor tendon sheath (Figure 5.8c)
- Finger held in slight flexion (Figure 5.8d)
- Pain with passive extension of the finger

## How do you manage infectious flexor tenosynovitis?

If caught early and in most cases, the FSI can be managed conservatively. This includes the following:

- Intravenous (IV) antibiotics – a broad spectrum antibiotic is started as per local policy
- Elevation – helps reduce swelling and pain
- Splinting – in early stages may not be needed, but in recovering stages

## Surgery

If, however, the patient is not responding to IV antibiotics within 24–48 hours, or presents late

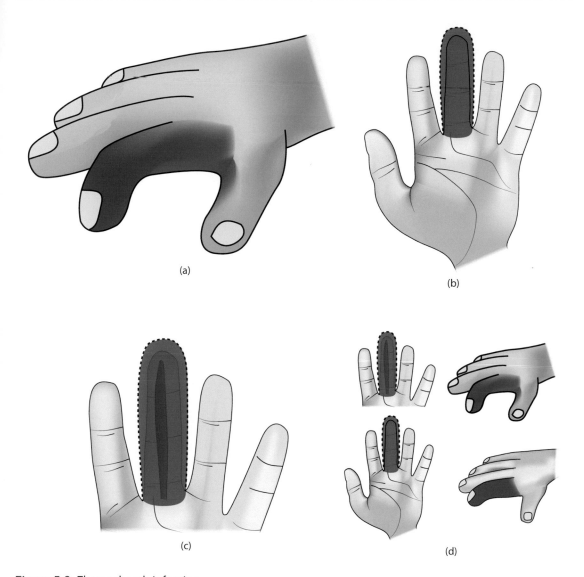

(a)

(b)

(c)

(d)

Figure 5.8 Flexor sheath infection.

with collection, a surgical intervention may be necessary. This then needs to be monitored and repeated washouts may be necessary.

Rehabilitation – hand therapy is initiated once FSI is under control.

## What are some of the complications of FSI infection?

FSI can cause significant damage to fingers and the hand if not identified early and managed appropriately. Common complications include stiffness and pain and can often lead to CRPS.

There is also risk of tendon rupture and in extreme cases loss of a finger.

Wrist pain is a common presentation in general practice. It may be sudden onset due to trauma or fall or can be insidious.

## What are the common causes of pain in wrist?

The cause of pain is very variable and it's important to know a few things. First, on which side is the pain located – is the pain radial or ulnar sided? Did it start acutely or over a period of time? Was there any injury?

Apart from fractures and sprain, the common causes of radial-sided wrist pain are de Quervain's disease, thumb arthritis, ganglion, scaphoid non-union advanced collapse (SNAC) or scapholunate advanced collapse (SLAC), Kienböck's disease, wrist arthritis, rheumatoid arthritis and osteoarthritis.

On the ulnar side, the common causes of pain include triangular fibrocartilage complex (TFCC) lesions, ulnar impingement, ganglion and tendinitis. Unusual causes include tumours around the tendons, nerve or bone.

## What symptoms or problems do these patients present with?

This depends on the dominance of hand and on which side the pain presents. Commonly patients present with difficulty in gripping objects, opening jars, twisting keys and other ADL.

## How do you diagnose the conditions?

After a detailed history, we perform an examination to see what the problem may be. This includes inspection, palpation and movements to investigate the problem and then arriving at a provisional diagnosis.

**Inspection:** Look for any swelling, deformity of joint or fingers and any features of widespread osteoarthritis. Look for muscle wasting, which may be the primary or secondary problem.

**Palpation:** Try and locate the tenderness, whether radial or ulnar, volar or dorsal. Check for tenderness in hand joints. Feel for any swelling to differentiate between bony or soft tissue.

**Movements:** Check for dorsiflexion and palmar flexion as well as radial and ulnar deviation. Check for supination and pronation – as a reduction could be because of wrist, forearm or elbow problems.

**Imaging:** Often we may need some diagnostic tests like plain radiographs, computed tomography (CT) scan or magnetic resonance imaging (MRI) scan to help with making a definitive diagnosis.

## How do you treat these patients?

There are non-surgical and surgical options.

## Non-surgical management

In the vast majority of cases, the initial treatment is non-operative, which involves simple analgesics like paracetamol or non-steroidal anti-inflammatory medication. This is often supplemented with a splint to support the painful joint. If this fails to help the symptoms the joint has, then a steroid injection can be performed. A steroid is a very powerful anti-inflammatory agent which helps reduce the pain and swelling in the joint.

## Surgical management

This is tailored to the underlying condition. It varies from doing key hole surgery to tidy up the joint to more definitive treatment in the form of release of the tendon sheath or removing the ganglion.

## Resources

1. www.gpnotebook.co.uk
2. www.patient.co.uk
3. www.medscape.com
4. www.orthobullets.com
5. http://www.us.elsevierhealth.com/greens-operative-hand-surgery-2-volume-set-9781455774272.html#panel1
6. www.kentorthpaedicpractice.co.uk

# 6

# Hip disorders

MATTHEW SEAH and VIKAS KHANDUJA

## Introduction

Hip pain is a common presenting complaint in primary care, with one study estimating the incidence of hip pain to be as high as 36%.[1] Femoroacetabular impingement (FAI), a recently described condition, now thought to be one of the major causes of hip pain in young adults, has an estimated incidence approaching 25%.[2] The differential diagnoses for hip and groin pain vary widely, including intra- and extra-articular hip pathology, as well as referred pain from other sources. Hip pathology also presents variably with groin, trochanteric, buttock, knee or thigh symptoms. The management of acute presentations such as trauma and infection are well described and here we review the diagnosis and initial management of several causes of hip pain, in particular, the newer and less easily diagnosed causes such as FAI and soft tissue problems in and around the hip. We draw from recent guidelines, the evidence in the literature and our own experience.

## What are the differential diagnoses of hip pain?

The aim of a focused history/examination is to confirm the hip as the source of pain. Additional laboratory tests and/or imaging and a diagnostic hip injection of local anaesthetic may be required to confirm that the source of the pain is the hip joint. Fractures, infection and avascular necrosis should be ruled out early, as they require prompt attention and treatment. Table 6.1 outlines all the causes for hip and groin pain and Table 6.2 outlines the systematic approach to history and examination for a patient presenting with hip and groin pain.

## How is a diagnosis made?

### History

- It is important to elicit a clear location of symptoms as patients variably refer to pain in the lower extremity and pelvic area as 'hip pain'.
- The patient should be specifically asked about the site of pain.
- Typically, intra-articular pathology presents with groin pain which may radiate to the knee

and/or the buttock. Pain in the thigh, buttocks or pain which radiates distal to the knee may originate from the spine or proximal thigh musculature.

- Onset/duration of symptoms is important, and past medical/surgical history should be explored, as well as the patient's social and recreational history.
- Intra-articular pathology may be associated with mechanical symptoms of locking, clicking and giving way, which should be elicited as well.

### Examination

- Include an analysis of the patient's gait (when they walk into the room, and observation of the patients' posture when standing or sitting) and assess for abductor function via the Trendelenburg test.
- Feel for specific points of tenderness – anterior superior iliac spine, pubic symphysis, greater trochanter and the ischial tuberosity. Check for tenderness over the adductors, abductors and flexors of the hip joint. Finally, check for a cough impulse in the inguinal and femoral region.
- Check the range of motion (ROM) of the joint (important to distinguish hip ROM from compensatory/complementary movement from the pelvis and lumbar spine). The normal ROM

Table 6.1 Causes of hip/groin pain

| Intra-articular | Extra-articular |
|---|---|
| Developmental dysplasia of the hip | Abductor/gluteal muscle tears |
| Legg–Calve–Perthes disease | Trochanteric bursitis |
| Slipped capital femoral epiphysis | Tendonitis (iliotibial band or iliopsoas) |
| Acetabular labral tears | Gluteal space syndrome |
| Ligamentum teres tears | Adductor tendonitis |
| Chondral flaps | Ischial bursitis |
| Pigmented villonodular synovitis (PVNS)/synovial chondromatosis | Hamstring tendinosis |
| Septic arthritis | Radicular pain (e.g. sciatica) |
| Osteomyelitis | Referred pain (e.g. from lumbar spine) |
| Osteoarthritis | Local nerve entrapment |
| Inflammatory arthropathy | Hernias (femoral and inguinal) |
| Femoroacetabular impingement (FAI) | Gynaecological and testicular pathology |
| Avascular necrosis of the femoral head | Stress fractures |
| Neoplastic | Subspinous syndrome |
| | Snapping hip syndromes |
| | Pubic symphysitis |

Table 6.2 Sensitivity and specificity of selected hip provocative tests

| Test/author | Sensitivity | Specificity | Positive likelihood ratio | Negative likelihood ratio |
|---|---|---|---|---|
| **FABER test – labral tears (if anterior groin pain); sacroiliac joint (SIJ) pathology (if pain over SIJ)** **Flexion, abduction and external rotation of the hip (Figure 6.2)** | | | | |
| Martin et al.[6] | 0.60 | 0.18 | 0.73 | 2.2 |
| **FADIR test – femoroacetabular impingement (FAI) – impingement test (anterior)** **Flexion, adduction and internal rotation of the hip** | | | | |
| Martin et al.[6] | 0.78 | 0.10 | 0.86 | 2.2 |
| **Impingement provocation test – posterior inferior labral tear** **(Patient prone) hyperextension, abduction and external rotation** | | | | |
| Leunig et al.[7] | 0.97 | 0.11 | 1.1 | 0.27 |
| **Stinchfield test – intra-articular pathology** **Straight leg raising against resistance** | | | | |
| Maslowski et al.[8] | 0.59 | 0.32 | 0.87 | 1.28 |

for hip flexion (tested with patient supine) is 110°–120°; the normal external and internal rotation are 40°–60° and 30°–40°, respectively (tested with patient supine with hip in 90° of flexion and knee in 90° of flexion) (Figure 6.1).

- Symptoms elicited at various points should be noted as hip pain throughout movement and suggests osteoarthritis (OA), while pain in certain positions or on specific provocative tests may point to another diagnosis.
- Various special tests have been described but the simplest is log rolling of the hip back and forth (leg in full extension on the examination couch). Log rolling moves only the femoral head in relation to the acetabulum and the surrounding capsule without significant excursion or stress on myotendinous structures or nerves. Absence of a positive log roll test does not preclude the hip as a source of symptoms but its presence greatly raises the suspicion. Active straight leg raising or straight leg raising against resistance often elicits hip symptoms. This manoeuver generates a large force across the articular surface.
- The sensitivity and specificity of some hip provocative tests are listed below.

- Finally, a thorough examination of the spine and knee along with the distal neurovascular status are essential to complete the examination.

## Imaging

- Standard weight-bearing anteroposterior (AP) radiographs of the pelvis and a cross-table lateral or frog lateral view of the hip are useful in diagnosing many causes of hip pain (Figure 6.3a and b).
- However, it should be noted that radiographs might not be sensitive to early degenerative disease. For example, in a series of 234 hips, Santori and Villar found arthroscopic evidence of OA in 32% of patients with normal radiographs.
- Magnetic resonance imaging (MRI) scans are essential for finally confirming the diagnosis of avascular necrosis, acetabular labral tears, chondral flaps and ligamentum teres tears.
- Ultrasound scans of the hip can be useful for diagnosing infection and aspirating fluid at the same time for confirmation of diagnosis and also for snapping syndromes in the non-acute situation.

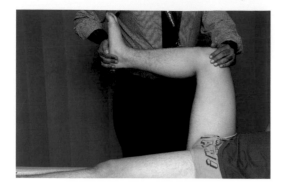

Figure 6.1 Measuring hip rotation in a patient.

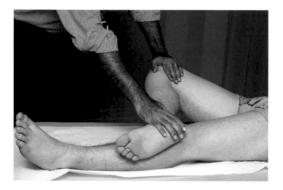

Figure 6.2 Performing the FABER test (flexion, abduction and external rotation of the hip).

- Computerised tomography (CT) scans of the hip are used to understand the morphology and as a preoperative planning tool in patients with dysplasia and FAI (Figure 6.4).

# What are some causes of hip pain in patients?

## Acute presentation

### Septic arthritis

Septic arthritis tends to occur in patients who are immune-compromised, or have had recent bacteraemia or intravenous drug abuse, recent trauma or comorbidities such as diabetes. This usually occurs in the acute setting and patients report systemic upset as well as swelling, erythema and heat over the affected joint, and painful active/passive ROM. Early diagnosis, antibiotic treatment and joint drainage (<48 hours) are required to preserve the articular cartilage.[2,3]

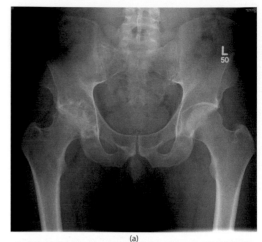

(a)

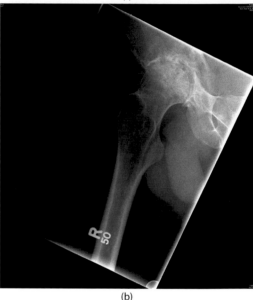

(b)

Figure 6.3 **(a)** AP radiograph of an osteoarthritic hip showing loss of joint space, subchondral sclerosis, osteophytosis and subchondral cysts and **(b)** lateral radiograph of the same hip.

### Avascular necrosis of the femoral head

This is associated with trauma, corticosteroid use, alcohol, smoking, systemic lupus erythematosus, sickle cell anaemia, storage disorders, coagulopathies and radiation treatment. No apparent cause is found in a fifth of patients. Patients report progressive stiffness and groin pain, and examination findings vary from normal in the early stages to a restricted ROM/antalgic gait in later stages consistent with degenerative OA. This condition needs

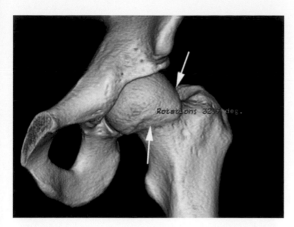

Figure 6.4 3D CT scan image showing the topography of a cam lesion and defining its margins (arrows).

to be picked up early for appropriate management and for avoiding further collapse of the femoral head and eventually degenerative changes. A high index of suspicion is necessary and a MRI scan clinches the diagnosis.

### Stress fractures

Stress fractures can either be fatigue fractures (repeated abnormal stresses on normal bone) or insufficiency fractures (physiological stress applied to abnormal bone). Patients typically present with activity-induced pain in the hip, groin, thigh or knee. Physical examination may be unspecific apart from diffuse pain localising to the hip or groin. Plain radiographs may be normal and a bone scan or an MRI scan is essential to confirm the diagnosis.

### Bone marrow oedema syndrome (transient osteoporosis of the hip)

This is characterised by gradual-onset hip pain with focal proximal femoral osteopenia on radiographs but improves over several months. MRI shows focal bone marrow oedema in the osteopenic areas, and patients tend to be young women in the third trimester of pregnancy or middle-aged men. Examination findings are often non-specific with pain elicited at extremes of ROM. The cause remains unknown, but many of these patients appear to be at risk of osteoporosis, and MRI findings are characteristic of trabecular bone injury. Nevertheless, management is conservative.

## Chronic presentation

### Osteoarthritis

The National Institute for Health and Care Excellence (NICE) has published guidelines on the diagnosis/management of OA in adults. OA is a common cause of morbidity in older adults. It is also seen in younger patients, where the disease may be at an earlier stage or be associated with conditions such as FAI. The prevalence of doctor-diagnosed hip OA in people aged <50 years approaches 1% according to a Swedish study. It is important to note that there is often a poor correlation between radiological appearances and symptoms: minimal degenerative changes can be associated with a lot of pain, and more dramatic radiological changes in joints can occur with minimal accompanying symptoms.

The NICE guidelines state that OA can be diagnosed clinically in a patient who (1) is above the age of 45 years, (2) has activity-related joint pain and (3) has either no morning joint-related stiffness or morning stiffness which lasts no longer than 30 minutes. An assessment should also be made of how symptoms affect the patient's function, quality of life, occupation, mood, relationships and leisure activities.

### Inflammatory arthritis

This comprises a number of systemic diseases which may involve the hip (e.g. rheumatoid arthritis and systemic lupus erythematosus). Joint pain is typically dull or progressive. Morning pain and stiffness (usually lasting more than an hour) are common and tend to improve with activity.

Prompt referral to a rheumatologist is indicated if there is persistent synovitis with an unknown cause (in small joints of the hands/feet; if more than one joint is affected). Local joint injections may relieve symptoms (but should not be prescribed prior to specialist assessment), while disease-modifying antirheumatic drugs (DMARDs) and the newer biologic agents are aimed at alleviating symptoms, slowing disease progression and preventing loss of function.

### Femoroacetabular impingement

FAI or hip impingement refers to production of pain when the femoral head neck junction abuts against the acetabular rim. This can happen because of morphological abnormalities on the acetabular or the femoral side. Two distinct types have been described and include the pincer or cam lesions, or a combination of both – the former is an acetabular (overcoverage) abnormality; cam lesions refer to asphericity of the femoral head. FAI has a strong association with subsequent OA and joint replacement.[3] Patients are often young and present with hip/groin pain and mechanical symptoms of locking or clicking. On examination, they often have positive impingement/FABER tests. Some patients have an exceptionally good ROM (e.g. ballet dancers, gymnasts or those with ligamentous laxity) and the impingement test is positive only in the extremes of internal rotation and flexion. They often report symptoms on leg hyperextension, as the hyperextended hip is in extreme internal rotation to the pelvis, and pain is produced. Once diagnosed, FAI can be managed effectively with arthroscopic surgery (Figures 6.5a and b, and 6.6), and there is enough literature reporting favourable short- to medium-term outcomes.[4]

### Acetabular labral tears

These were initially described in patients with hip dysplasia and OA, and subsequently in Perthes disease, trauma and FAI. Patients report dull/sharp groin pain (occasionally buttock pain) of variable onset, and mechanical symptoms such as painful clicking.[3] Symptoms are exacerbated by activity and impingement test often elicits symptoms.

Radiographs may show early degenerative changes or associated pathology (e.g. hip dysplasia, FAI, acetabular anteversion/retroversion). Diagnosis is made with MR arthrography (sensitivity >90%, specificity 100%). If patients fail to respond to conservative treatment, hip arthroscopy (Figures 6.7a and b) can be offered with good short-term results reported for both labral debridement and repair.

### Loose bodies

Intra-articular loose bodies are frequently associated with other pathology, such as posttrauma, OA, avascular necrosis of the femoral head, osteochondritis dissecans, synovial chondromatosis or pigmented villonodular synovitis (PVNS). Symptomatic onset is dependent on the underlying pathology, and patients report groin pain/mechanical symptoms.

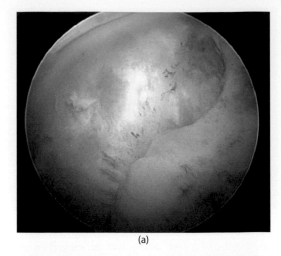

(a)

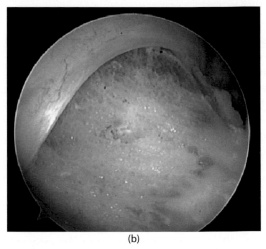

(b)

Figure 6.5 Head/neck junction of the hip **(a)** prior to and **(b)** following cam excision.

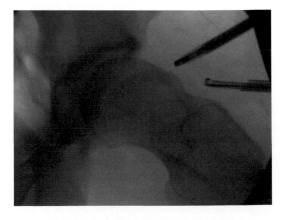

Figure 6.6 Extended neck lateral hip fluoroscopic image showing the cam deformity.

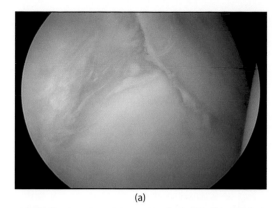

(a)

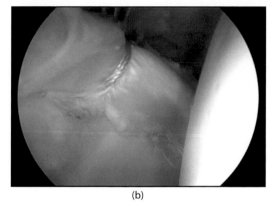

(b)

Figure 6.7 Impingement lesion at hip arthroscopy **(a)** before and **(b)** following repair.

Radiographs/CT can identify ossified/osteochondral loose bodies, but MRI may be required to identify cartilaginous loose bodies and potential synovial or soft tissue pathology. Symptomatic intra-articular loose bodies may damage joint cartilage and arthroscopy is therefore useful in suitable patients.

### Ligamentum teres injury

These are often associated with other pathology: complete tears with hip dislocation, partial tears with a subacute event and degenerative tears with joint pathology. Symptoms may include mechanical symptoms such as popping, locking or giving way. Examination findings are usually not pathognomonic but should identify an intra-articular source of symptoms. Most of them are treated conservatively, but arthroscopy can be helpful in relieving patients with persistent mechanical symptoms. In some patients, especially athletes and gymnasts, instability can be a problem and ligamentum teres reconstruction has been carried out successfully in this cohort.

### Snapping hip syndrome

Patients usually present with a history of a painful (and frequently audible) snap when the hip is brought through certain movements. Three variations exist: (1) the iliotibial band (ITB) rubbing over the greater trochanter; (2) the iliopsoas tendon rubbing over the femoral head or anterior hip structures (e.g. iliopectineal eminence) and (3) snapping sensations secondary to intra-articular pathology (e.g. acetabular labral tear or chondral fragments). Symptoms felt laterally tend to suggest extra-articular causes, while intra-articular causes (2 and 3) tend to cause groin pain. In cases of external snapping, when the ITB rubs over the greater trochanter, trochanteric bursitis may result, and pain is elicited on direct palpation over the bursa. Snapping can often be reproduced with the patients lying on their side as the hip is brought from flexion to extension.

Dynamic ultrasound can demonstrate the snapping ITB and associated bursitis/tendinopathy and also iliopsoas snapping in cases of internal snapping.[5] Trochanteric bursitis and external snapping hip are generally managed conservatively and a local anaesthetic/steroid injection into the bursa can be both diagnostic and therapeutic.[5] Surgical release (arthroscopic or open) is rarely required for recalcitrant cases. As far as internal or iliopsoas snapping is concerned, most cases can be managed conservatively as well with ultrasound-guided injections and physiotherapy which is aimed at stretching the iliopsoas tendon. In some cases where conservative management fails, arthroscopic release of the iliopsoas tendon provides good results.

### Adductor tendinopathy

This is a common cause of hip pain in athletes, especially in sports with repetitive kicking, quick starts or direction changes. Patients typically report groin/medial thigh pain of variable onset, with tenderness along the adductors and painful resisted adduction. Diagnosis is made clinically, but ultrasound/MRI shows characteristic features.

Management is mainly conservative. Injections at the adductor longus enthesis can be considered if patients do not respond to initial management.

### Hip abductor pathology

Analogous to rotator cuff injury, tendinopathy and acute/degenerate tears of the gluteus minimus and medius may occur. Patients present with dull lateral hip pain, focal tenderness at the gluteal insertion and occasionally with weak hip abduction. Plain radiographs may show calcification at the tendon insertion but ultrasound may be more useful for diagnosis. Management is conservative but some cases do require surgical intervention to repair the tears.

## Athletic pubalgia/sports hernia

The aetiology is unknown, but injury to the rectus insertion on the pubic symphysis has been implicated and has also been described as an occult hernia through the posterior inguinal wall without a clinically recognisable hernia. 'Gilmore's groin' refers to injury to the external oblique aponeurosis and conjoint tendon, with dehiscence between the conjoint tendon and inguinal ligament. There may be a higher incidence in sports requiring repetitive twisting, and in athletes with pronounced muscular imbalance between strong thigh muscles and weaker abdominal muscles (greater shearing forces across the symphysis).

Patients report gradual-onset, activity-associated pain (in the adductors, perineum, rectus or testicular areas) which is relieved with rest. Management is conservative initially, and if there is no improvement in symptoms then surgical intervention in terms of the repair of the hernia is indicated.

## Osteitis pubis

First described in patients who underwent suprapubic surgery, this now describes pathologies which affect the pubic symphysis and surrounding muscular insertions. Patients report sharp/achy anterior pelvic pain which radiates to the adductors or lower abdomen. Palpation of the symphysis or rising from a seated position is painful.

Plain radiography in acute cases may appear normal, while chronic cases may reveal cystic changes, sclerosis or narrowing/widening at the symphysis. Management is conservative, and local injection may be diagnostic/therapeutic. Surgery is infrequently performed and the long-term outcomes remain unknown.

# Nerve entrapment syndromes

## Deep gluteal syndrome

Classically described as the **piriformis syndrome**, the terminology has now been changed to deep gluteal syndrome and encompasses entrapment of the sciatic nerve in the gluteal region. The sciatic nerve emerges from the greater sciatic notch inferior to the piriformis and its compression may cause posterior thigh pain. This can be caused by trauma, piriformis hypertrophy/spasm or anatomical variations. Patients report pain over the sacroiliac joint (SIJ)/sciatic notch and in the sciatic nerve distribution. Prolonged sitting exacerbates symptoms, while walking tends to relieve pain. Symptoms can be elicited with resisted abduction/adduction with the hip in flexion/internal rotation. In contrast to radicular causes of sciatica, straight leg raising frequently does not reproduce symptoms.

Management is conservative and ultrasound- or MR-guided injections may be diagnostic/therapeutic. Surgical release has been reported with good short-term results.

## Meralgia paraesthetica

Compression of the lateral femoral cutaneous nerve results in pain or altered sensation of the lateral aspect of the thigh. Associated factors include obesity, diabetes, previous pelvic surgery and tight clothing/waist straps (e.g. tool belts). Tinel's sign may be elicited 1 cm medial and inferior to the anterior superior iliac spine. Most cases settle with conservative management, but in some cases, surgical release is required and produces good results.

## Ilioinguinal nerve compression

The ilioinguinal nerve can be compressed with abdominal muscle hypertrophy, pregnancy or less frequently, previous bone graft harvesting. Symptoms are usually felt in the inguinal region with radiation to the genitalia. Tinel's sign may be elicited 3 cm inferior and medial to the anterior superior iliac spine, and hip hyperextension may provoke symptoms.

## Obturator nerve compression

This is associated with previous pelvic procedures or pelvic masses and presents with a medial thigh pain or numbness which is exacerbated by activity and relieved with rest. Pain can be elicited by external rotation and adduction of the hip while the patient stands. There may also be associated weakness of the adductors.

## How do I inject the trochanteric bursa?

The trochanteric bursa is located over the lateral prominence of the greater trochanter of the femur. Palpating the femur proximally and laterally identifies the greater trochanter, and the injection site is the point of maximal tenderness and/or swelling.

With the patient in the lateral recumbent position (affected side facing the ceiling), the skin is cleaned with antiseptic solution. A combination of local anaesthetic and steroid is injected via a 22- or 25-gauge needle, inserted perpendicular to the skin. The needle should be inserted directly down to bone and then withdrawn 2–3 mm before aspirating to ensure that the needle is not in a vessel and then injecting. A longer needle may be required in obese patients (Figure 6.8).

Remember that up to three bursae, arranged around the greater trochanter in a triangular configuration, can be affected.

Figure 6.8 Line diagram showing approach for trochanteric bursa injection.

## Are there any associated risks?

The risk of hyperglycaemia in patients with diabetes is very small and transient, even for longer acting corticosteroid preparations. Adrenal suppression from intra-articular corticosteroids has been described but usually lasts less than 2 weeks when it occurs. Other potential risks include skin hypopigmentation, fat atrophy, tendon rupture and facial flushing.

Injection should be avoided across suspected cellulitis, in areas of infectious arthritis or bursitis, in patients with bacteraemia or in severely immunocompromised patients. In particular, the injection of joints which contain prosthetic hardware should be avoided; and patients with such prosthetic hardware should be referred to an orthopaedic surgeon.

## When does a patient need referral to secondary care?

Appropriate history, examination and investigations are important to exclude childhood hip disorders, trauma and infection. When the patient fails to respond to conservative management, specialist referral should be considered. This young adult patient group has high demands, and both diagnosis and management of pathology in this group can be difficult. The literature is insufficiently robust to draw firm conclusions regarding best practices for some conditions, and much work remains to be done to consolidate the role of the newer surgical interventions. Therefore, if in doubt, it is best to refer patients in this age group for a specialist opinion earlier on in their presentation.

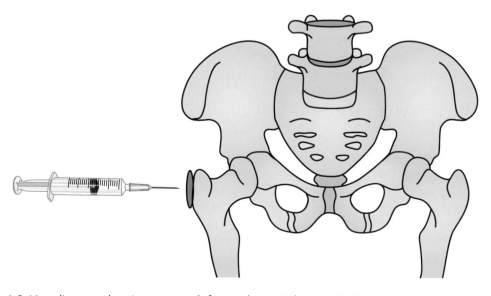

Figure 6.8 Line diagram showing approach for trochanteric bursa injection.

## What information should a patient be given prior to referral for joint replacement?

The NICE guidelines recommend that when discussing the possibility of joint surgery, check that the patients have been offered at least the core treatments for OA (e.g. patient educational material, interventions to achieve weight loss if the patient is overweight, etc.) and give them information about:

- The benefits and risks of surgery and the potential consequences of not having surgery
- Recovery and rehabilitation after surgery
- How having a prosthesis might affect them
- How care pathways are organised in the local area

## Infection following a total hip replacement – what should I be concerned about?

If you suspect that the patient has an infection associated with the joint procedure, especially in the first few weeks following surgery, the orthopaedic team should be contacted urgently. An infection should be suspected when:

- The wound starts to leak fluid having been dry or continues to leak fluid beyond 7 days after the procedure.
- Part of or the entire wound becomes swollen, red or sore to touch.
- There is sudden increase in pain around the patient's hip and he or she feels shivery and/or unwell.
- Pain which fails to settle following surgery or pain which develops some time later can be caused by infection, and in these cases, the wound can remain normal.

## What should I look for in the postoperative radiographs following a hip replacement?

The postoperative radiograph (Figure 6.9) is often a prerequisite before the patient's discharge. Subsequent follow-up radiographs form part of the ongoing assessment of a prosthetic joint, and changes in the appearance of the components and surrounding bone are of significant diagnostic

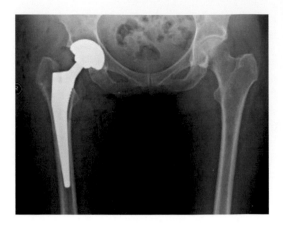

Figure 6.9 Postoperative radiograph showing a right uncemented total hip replacement. Parameters which can be assessed include leg length, centre of rotation, acetabular component inclination, femoral stem positioning, acetabular component anteversion (on lateral radiograph) and cement mantle quality (in cemented prostheses).

value. Short-term complications, which are evident on radiographs, are mainly issues of component malposition and adequacy of fixation. Long-term complications are centred on component loosening, infection or fracture. Radiological findings, which should prompt urgent orthopaedic referral, include:

- Gross component malposition
- Periprosthetic lucency > 2 mm or progressive changes
- Cement fracture
- Dislocation
- Periprosthetic fracture

## What are the reasons for needing a revision hip replacement?

A revision hip replacement may be required for the following reasons:

- The implant may become painful due to wear and loosening (e.g. thigh pain due to a loosening femoral stem and movement in the femoral canal).
- Total hip replacements (THRs) can dislocate on repeated occasions, and revision surgery may be needed in cases of repeat dislocation.
- Patients may fall and sustain a periprosthetic fracture.

- If a deep infection develops, revision surgery will frequently be required to eradicate the infection and to implant new non-infected components. A single operation may be performed to eradicate the infection (single-stage revision), but often surgeons prefer to do a two-stage revision involving two separate operations.

## SUMMARY POINTS

- Hip pain in young adults should not be ignored.
- Appropriate history, examination and imaging (and laboratory tests where appropriate) are important to exclude childhood hip disorders, trauma and infection.
- Symptoms and signs may be difficult to elicit in patients who normally put their hips at extremes of ROM (e.g. martial artists, gymnasts, climbers).
- Look for reduced internal rotation in 90° of flexion and a positive impingement test.
- Commence a trial of analgesia, physical therapy/activity modification and keep under follow-up.
- Normal radiographs do not exclude early degenerative change in the joint.
- Consider specialist referral if symptoms persist for more than 3 months or worsen.

## Ongoing research

- Following the successful development of joint registries (for patients who have had joint replacements), hip arthroscopy registers are currently being developed in several countries (e.g. UK, Sweden).
- Arthroscopic intervention for FAI produces good short-term results but it remains to be seen whether it actually changes the natural history of the OA.
- As articular cartilage has little capacity for healing, joint-preserving surgical techniques are continuously being developed (e.g. autologous chondrocyte transplantation, mosaicplasty, osteochondral allograft transplantation and stem cell implantation).

## Resources for patients

The musculoskeletal zone (NHS Inform) has been developed with the help of patients, physiotherapists and doctors to bring together the best possible information and advice for preventing, treating and recovering from musculoskeletal disorders at home and in the workplace. http://www.nhsinform.co.uk/MSK/lowerbody/hip

## References

1. Murphy LB, Helmick CG, Schwartz TA, Renner JB, Tudor G, Koch GG et al. One in four people may develop symptomatic hip osteoarthritis in his or her lifetime. *Osteoarthritis Cartilage.* 2010;18(11):1372–1379.
2. Monazzam S, Bomar JD, Dwek JR, Hosalkar HS, Pennock AT. Development and prevalence of femoroacetabular impingement-associated morphology in a paediatric and adolescent population: A CT study of 225 patients. *Bone Joint J.* 2013;95-B(5):598–604.
3. Imam S, Khanduja V. Current concepts in the management of femoroacetabular impingment. *Int Orthop.* 2011 Oct;35(10):1427–1435.
4. Bedi A, Kelly BT, Khanduja V. Arthroscopic hip preservation surgery: Current concepts and perspective. *Bone Joint J.* 2013 Jan;95-B(1):10–19.
5. Del Buono A, Papalia R, Khanduja V, Denaro V, Maffulli N. Management of the greater trochanteric pain syndrome: A systematic review. *Br Med Bull.* 2012 Jun;102:115–131.
6. Martin RL, Irrgang JJ, Sekiya JK. The diagnostic accuracy of a clinical examination in determining intra-articular hip pain for potential hip arthroscopy candidates. *Arthroscopy.* 2008;24(9):1013–1018.
7. Leunig M, Werlen S, Ungersbock A, Ito K, Ganz R. Evaluation of the acetabular labrum by MR arthrography. *J Bone Joint Surg Br.* 1997;79(2):230–234.
8. Maslowski E, Sullivan W, Forster HJ, Gonzalez P, Kaufman M, Vidal A et al. The diagnostic validity of hip provocation maneuvers to detect intra-articular hip pathology. *PM R.* 2010;2(3):174–181.

# 7

# Knee disorders

SANJEEV ANAND and TIM GREEN

## Introduction

Problems affecting the knee joint are the second most common cause of musculoskeletal presentation to a general practice clinic. These problems can present in an acute setting or as chronic long-term conditions affecting quality of life and leading to disability.

## Acute soft tissue knee injuries

Acute knee injuries leading to fractures around the knee joint are unlikely to present to a general practice clinic. Because of difficulty in weight bearing and catastrophic presentation, most patients present themselves to emergency departments and get diagnosed appropriately. Acute 'soft tissue' injuries of the knee are, however, frequently missed and patients may present to their general practitioner due to persistent concerns.

Acute 'soft tissue' knee injuries are commonly associated with sports and young active people. It should not be forgotten that there are also significant injuries which affect the older and less active age group. Early identification of these injuries allows for early diagnosis, counselling and appropriate rehabilitation to prevent prolonged morbidity, secondary cartilaginous or meniscus damage. Unfortunately, diagnosis can be missed or delayed by clinicians across many specialties including orthopaedic surgery.[1] The first encounter by a clinician is the best time to identify the severity of the injury and refer the patient, so that an appropriate management plan can be initiated.

## Why is the knee joint vulnerable to injuries?

The knee joints are covered only by a thin layer of soft tissue and bear the weight of the whole body above them. Although it is a hinge joint with primarily flexion–extension movement, it also allows rotatory movements. The joint stability is provided mainly by soft tissues rather than significant bony structures. The primary stabilisers are the ligaments: the anterior cruciate ligament (ACL), posterior cruciate ligament (PCL), lateral collateral ligament (LCL), medial collateral ligament (MCL) and posterolateral corner (PLC), providing support in translations, angulations and rotations. The crescent- and wedge-shaped medial and lateral menisci increase the depth and contact surface area for the femoral condyles and allow rotatory movement on top of the tibia plateau. A congruent and healthy cartilage allows painless and functional range of movements. The joint capsule provides the remaining stability. An injury to any of these structures may disturb the homeostasis of the knee.[2]

## How do I identify patients needing referral to secondary service following an acute knee injury?

### History

Almost every 'soft tissue' injury to the knee has its typical history. The meniscus is usually injured by a twisting grinding force with the knee in flexion, e.g. deep squatting position. The patient will experience acute pain. If the meniscus displaces and gets lodged between the tibia and femur, the knee will be painfully locked (inability to fully extend). Swelling is often noticeable hours later. ACL injury is commonly due to a sudden deceleration and pivoting force on the knee (e.g. rapid change of direction while running). If the injury is caused by contact, it is due to a valgus or hyperextension force. The patient reports an audible painful pop and inability to continue with activity. Swelling is immediate, in contrast to meniscus injury. The mechanism of patellar dislocation

is not dissimilar to ACL injury, but the patient reports the knee 'dislocates' with sudden collapse. Swelling is immediate with pain in the medial side of the knee.[2]

*A very useful predictor of a significant soft tissue knee injury is the history of knee swelling after an injury. Knee swelling following a traumatic injury is a result of bleeding in the joint (haemarthrosis) and should be regarded as a serious injury until proven otherwise.* The common causes of painful traumatic knee swelling in the general population are (Table 7.1) intra-articular ligament injuries (40%–45%), patellar dislocation (8%–25%) and meniscus injuries (10%–32%). ACL rupture represents almost half of the ligamentous injury.[1,2]

Although this section's focus is on these three injuries, there are other significant 'soft tissue' injuries which will be briefly mentioned here. The classical dashboard injury where a posterior force is applied to the tibia relative to the femur in knee flexion or hyperflexion knee injury from a fall is associated with PCL injury. Rupture of the extensor knee tendons (quadriceps tendon and patellar tendon) occurs following a forced eccentric contraction of the quadriceps muscle (muscle forced to lengthen in contraction) with the knee in some flexion.

History taking should be completed by asking for the previous function of the affected knee. Open- and closed-ended questions should be used judiciously. Is it the first injury? Is there coexisting arthritis that is inflammatory, crystal or degenerative in nature? Was there any problem or pain in the knee prior to the current presentation? Medication such as warfarin can cause spontaneous haemarthrosis or worsen intra-articular bleeding. The quinolones antibiotics and steroid abuse are infamously associated with tendon rupture. Occupation, social and systemic medical history can assist in the decision making of management of the injured knee.[2]

Table 7.1 Causes of painful traumatic knee swelling

| Causes | % |
| --- | --- |
| Ligament injury | 40–45 |
| Patellar dislocation | 8–25 |
| Meniscus injury | 10–32 |
| Others | 15–25 |

*Source:* Lee L et al., *Sage*, 7, 428–436, 2014.

## Examination

Physical examination of a patient with acute knee injury is usually hindered by the patient's pain and restricted range of movement, but it is possible to elicit the cause of the pain to guide appropriate investigation or management. The role of clear communication to the patient during examination of an injured knee is absolutely crucial. This will prepare the patient in anticipation of the clinician's probing.

Observing the gait or posture of the patient should provide the clinician with some idea whether there are also additional problems apart from the knee. Persistent difficulty in weight bearing on the affected limb would suggest significant injury. Varus thrust is indicative of injury to posterolateral ligaments. There is subluxation of the knee with varus deformity when one bears weight on the affected knee due to the incompetent PLC structures. The presence of bruising can hint towards contact injury. Injury to intra-articular structures (ACL, PCL, meniscus tears, osteochondral injuries) would cause bleeding and swelling limited to the knee joint while injury to extra-articular structures (MCL, LCL, PLC) can cause diffuse bruising and swelling in relation to the anatomical location of the concerned ligament (Figure 7.1).[2]

Palpate the affected limb by starting away from and working towards the knee, e.g. foot and ankle or mid-thigh, to reassure the patient and also to simultaneously check for other injury. Moving carefully towards the knee, the clinician can begin to locate the 'lighthouse' landmarks or tibial tuberosity and patella (Figure 7.2). From the tibial tuberosity, the digit or thumb is moved superiorly to feel the continuity of longitudinal band-like structure of patella tendon to the bony inferior apex of patella. The 'soft spots' lateral and medial to the patella tendon lead to the lateral and medial joint lines, respectively. Tenderness along the joint line suggests meniscus injury.[2]

Proximal to the patella, the continuity of the quadriceps tendon is also examined. This can be better appreciated by asking the patient to actively extend the knee or to press the knee down against examination table to fully extend the knee. Swelling and a palpable gap along the quadriceps and patellar tendons above and below the patella, respectively, suggests tendon rupture.

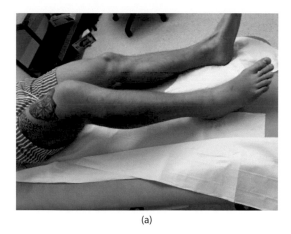

(a)

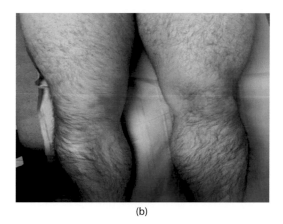

(b)

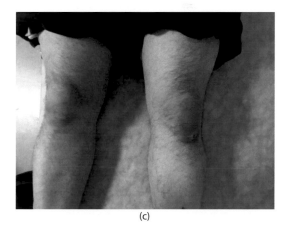

(c)

Figure 7.1 (a) Bruising after injury suggests capsular injury. (b) Right knee intra-articular swelling obliterating parapatellar fossae. (c) Prepatellar bursitis in left knee showing anterior extra-articular inflammation with no intraarticular swelling.

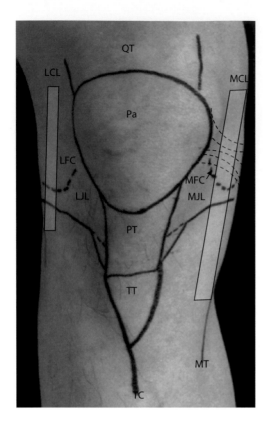

Figure 7.2 Surface anatomy of the knee. QT, quadriceps tendon; Pa, patella; LFC, lateral femoral condyle; MFC, medial femoral condyle; LJL, lateral joint line; MJL, medial joint line; PT, patella tendon; TT, tibial tuberosity; TC, tibial crest (anterior tibial border); MT, medial tibial border; curved dashed lines, medial patellofemoral ligament; LCL, lateral collateral ligament (schematic); MCL, medial collateral ligament (schematic).

Following acute patellar dislocation, examination will reveal tenderness along the injured medial restraint of the patella or the medial patellofemoral ligament (MPFL). The MPFL originates on the medial the femoral condyle, between the medial femoral epicondyle and the adductor tubercle. It courses laterally to attach to the medial aspect of patella. Tenderness at the inferomedial patella border and lateral femoral condyle are consistent with traumatic tangential patellar displacement causing chondral damage. Attempted lateral displacement of the patella by the clinician or the 'apprehension test' will reproduce pain and the uncomfortable sensation of a dislocating patella (Figure 7.3).[2]

Any asymmetry including loss of the parapatellar groove indicates an effusion or haemarthrosis (Figure 7.1b). Severe swelling can be demonstrated

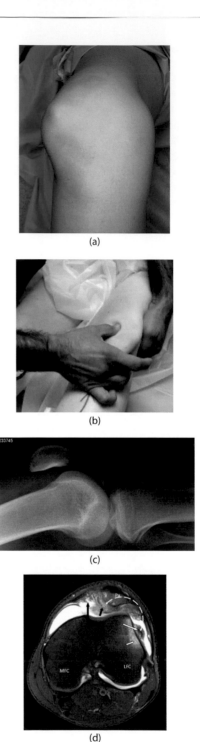

Figure 7.3 Acute patella dislocation. **(a)** Clinical picture showing lateral patella displacement. **(b)** Look for apprehension on attempted lateral subluxation of patella. **(c)** Plain x-ray showing small flake of bone representing significant osteochondral injury. **(d)** MR scan showing mechanism of patella dislocation l/t rupture of MPFL and osteochondral fracture resulting from re-entry injury.

by performing patellar tap – firm downward pressure on the patella to elicit palpable tap of a ballotable patella against the trochlea of the femur. This should not be mistaken for prepatellar bursitis, which is extra-articular, and the swelling lies directly over the patella (Figure 7.1c). In a more subtle knee swelling or effusion, the sweep test can be performed by placing a palm just proximal to the patella and with the other hand, 'sweeping' the medial side of the knee to empty the area of any fluid followed by a lateral pressure while observing for a bulge over the medial side indicating presence of effusion.

Check for range of movement of the knee. It is helpful to start at the end of examination table, holding both heels to assess extension of the knee

(Figure 7.4a). Hyperextension suggests posterior capsule or PLC injury. The knee is usually in a position of comfort, which is slight flexion due to pain and swelling. Encourage the patient to extend the knee actively. Inability to actively extend the knee from a flexed position may suggest disruption of extensor mechanism – one trick is for the physician to place a palm behind the knee and asking the patient to press down onto the palm or examination table. A meniscus tear with displaced bucket handle pattern can cause locked knee with an inability to extend the knee both actively or passively.[2] This will most likely require surgical intervention.

Further examinations are required to assess stability of the knee. It can be difficult to assess for ACL or

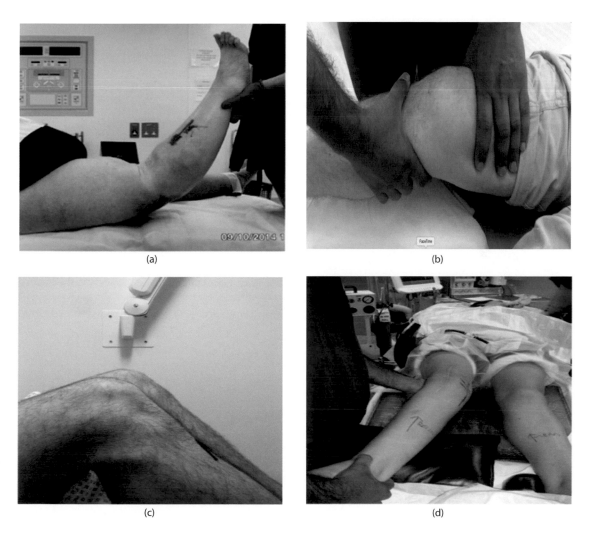

(a)

(b)

(c)

(d)

Figure 7.4 Ligament assessment. **(a)** Increased passive hyperextension suggests posterior capsular and posterolateral corner injury. **(b)** Lachman test for ACL laxity. **(c)** Posterior tibial sag suggesting PCL injury. **(d)** Assessing collateral stability.

PCL injury in an acutely swollen knee. The Lachman test (Figure 7.4b) is a commonly used test to detect ACL tear, followed by the anterior drawer test. Usually, this is better tolerated a few days after injury. Assess the PCL first from standing by the side of patient with both knees flexed to about 90° with the heels at the same level. Check for the symmetry of the level of tibia tuberosity – posterior sag of the affected knee may be obvious in PCL injury (Figure 7.4c).[2]

Assessment of an acutely injured knee is not complete without checking for the integrity of collateral ligaments to further determine the degree of stability and requirement for urgent surgical opinion. Palpate the MCLs, which is a broad flat band coursing from the medial femoral epicondyle to the medial tibial condyle and the LCL, which courses from the lateral femoral epicondyle to the head of the fibula (Figure 7.2). Tenderness indicates a possible injury. One hand holds the lower leg above the ankle, while the other applies valgus or varus force at a slightly flexed knee to check for MCL and LCL stability, respectively. Collateral stability can be graded as Grade 1 (less than 5 mm joint opening); Grade 2 (5–10 mm joint opening) and Grade 3 (more than 10 mm opening or no end point). Isolated Grade 1 and 2 injuries can be managed non-operatively. Grade 3 collateral ligament injuries are considered unstable and may require

surgery.[2] The presence of medial and lateral laxity in an acutely injured swollen knee would suggest a multiligamentous injury, which needs urgent attention in a specialist unit (Figure 7.4d).

Severe knee injuries can be complicated by neurovascular injury. It would be very unlikely that a patient with neurovascular injury would present for assessment after a few days, but neurovascular examination is good clinical practice.[2]

Salient history and typical physical examination findings in a patient with knee injury, are summarised in Table 7.2.

## Anterior cruciate ligament

ACL injury can happen in isolation or in combination with other ligaments or structures indicating more severe injury compromising the stability and function of the knee. ACL injury commonly occurs in late adolescence. There is a higher incidence in men, but interestingly studies have reported that females participating in similar pivoting and jumping activities are 2–9 times more at risk of suffering from ACL injury. There are different aetiological hypotheses for this increased risk in women. First, ligaments are laxer in women due to the influence of female hormones, making a female knee joint 'looser' and predisposing it to injury. Second, there

Table 7.2 Salient history and typical physical examination findings in knee injury

| | Anterior cruciate ligament (ACL) | Meniscal injury | Patella dislocation |
|---|---|---|---|
| Mechanism of injury | Sudden change in direction of the knee and body with the foot as a pivot | Twisting injury with knee in flexion (e.g. squatting position) | Many similarities to ACL or meniscal injury Less commonly from direct trauma |
| Patient's description | Painful 'pop' in the knee | Locking or inability to extend knee due to a 'block resistance' requires urgent referral | May have witnessed dislocated patella |
| Knee swelling | Immediate | Hours/next day | Degree of swelling correlates to severity |
| Examination | Lachman Anterior drawer | Effusion (small to moderate amount of swelling) with joint line tenderness | If unreduced, patella located lateral to knee with inability to extend Tenderness of medial knee restraint Patella apprehension test |

Source: Lee L et al., *Sage*, 7, 428–436, 2014.

is an anatomical difference in the bony structure of the knee joint in women. The femoral intercondylar notch is narrower in women, which subjects the ACL to increased stress during twisting or pivoting movements. Also, difference in landing posture after a jump makes women more prone to ACL injury.[3]

ACL injuries are usually non-contact injuries and often happen following hyperextension, quick deceleration or rotational injuries. Patients give a history of sudden pain with a popping sensation and collapse of the leg in the middle of a game. This is followed by rapid swelling of the knee, which indicates haemarthrosis. The knee can remain painful and swollen for a few weeks. Once the acute symptoms settle, patients typically complain of the knee 'giving way' on sudden cutting manoeuvres or change of direction, which typically limit their ability to participate in physical activities. Occasionally, patients would very graphically demonstrate their feeling of instability with a 'double fist sign', with two rotating fists on top of each other, simulating a grinding motion of the knee joint. A positive Lachman or anterior drawer test would confirm the diagnosis (Figure 7.4b).[2]

Plain x-rays may occasionally show a small flake of bone at the outer edge of the lateral tibial plateau

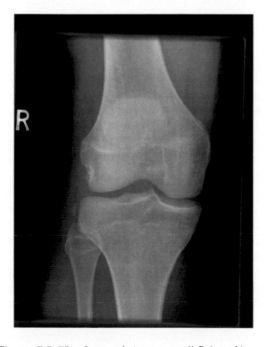

Figure 7.5 The Segond sign, a small flake of bone visible on the lateral aspect of the proximal tibia, is suggestive of ACL injury.

(Segond sign) (Figure 7.5). Presence of this fracture is very suggestive of ACL injury and should not be ignored. Magnetic resonance imaging (MRI) scan, if available, helps to aid and confirm clinical impression. In the absence of knee swelling or any objective clinical findings, it may be reasonable to withhold MRI scan unless symptoms are persistent. However, in the presence of significant knee swelling, an urgent MRI scan would be useful to rule out any significant injury.

All patients with suspected ACL injury should be referred as per local protocol for further assessment, appropriate further investigation, rehabilitation and counselling. In isolated ACL injury, a knee immobiliser is unnecessary. Patients may be offered crutches for a limited time, while initial pain and discomfort settle. Referral to physiotherapy should be performed immediately to maintain range of movement and develop quadriceps strength. In an active person, consider an early referral to an orthopaedic surgeon. Patients whose sports or work involve pivoting while weight bearing on the affected limb are more likely to require surgery to allow return to an acceptable level of function. However, not all ACL injuries in an active young person would require surgery. In a randomised study involving young active adults with ACL injury, the 5-year outcomes were similar in the early reconstructive surgery group as compared to rehabilitation and an optional delayed reconstruction group.[4]

Although ACL reconstruction is not protective against the development of osteoarthritis, delay in appropriate rehabilitation or surgery can potentially cause further internal damage to the cartilage and meniscus due to repeated giving way of the knee. Surgery is indicated for patients with recurrent instability from an ACL-deficient knee – that is with a history of the knee giving way, on sudden turning, or pivoting while weight bearing on affected leg.

## Acute patella dislocation

Acute traumatic patella dislocation is more common in the younger population, women or those involved in rigorous physical activity for example military recruits. Articular cartilage injury has been reported in up to 95% of patients following an episode of acute patella dislocation.[5] This injury to articular cartilage happens as the dislocated patella reduces back to its natural position. As the patella returns back, the medial edge of the patella hits the lateral edge of the lateral femoral condyle causing articular injury. Occasionally, this may result in shearing off a large piece of articular cartilage from the joint surface. It is important to identify this injury, as an early surgery to fix these detached fragments has potential to restore normal joint surface. X-rays may show thin slivers of bone in joint and should not be ignored as inconsequential. This thin bony sliver, visible on x-ray, represents the radiopaque portion of a large articular cartilage fragment, which would not otherwise be visible on plain x-rays (Figure 7.3c). The presence of large haemarthrosis with or without visible osteochondral fragment on x-rays suggests significant injury needing urgent MRI scan and specialist opinion.

Acute patella dislocation can be due to contact or non-contact injury. It is almost always a lateral dislocation with the knee in either extension or flexion with valgus stress to the knee or external rotation of the foot. There are often many similarities between the mechanism of injury leading to patella dislocation and ACL rupture. Acute patella dislocation would quite often spontaneously reduce as the patient extends his/her knee after the injury. At other times, acute dislocation may have been reduced by paramedics or in the accident and emergency (A&E) department. Unless the patella is seen in the dislocated position at the time of initial injury, history alone cannot always distinguish a patellar dislocation which has reduced spontaneously from an ACL rupture. It is important as part of history to enquire about previous patellofemoral joint symptoms, instability or dislocations. Clinically, patients would have bruising and pain over the medial aspect of the patella and knee joint. The 'apprehension test' as described earlier is likely to be positive (Figure 7.3b).[2]

A skyline view of the knee is always requested, along with routine anteroposterior (AP) and lateral views. The skyline view shows the patellofemoral morphology, alignment and presence of fractures following patella dislocation. Fat-fluid level indicating lipohaemarthrosis from intra-articular fracture or any small flake of bone seen within the joint in plain x-rays may signify significant osteochondral injury and should not be ignored (Figure 7.3c). An MRI scan would help confirm the diagnosis.[2]

In acute traumatic patella dislocation without any fracture provide analgesia and immobilisation using a well-fitted knee splint in slight flexion, for comfort after reduction. This is followed by prompt physiotherapy to encourage weight bearing and mobilisation.

There is high reported incidence (40%–50%) of recurrent patella dislocation after an initial episode. The risk factors for patellar redislocation are personal or family history of patellar dislocations, soft tissue and bony abnormalities such as hyperlaxity of joints and medial quadriceps weakness, femoral trochlear dysplasia, lower limb malalignment or high riding patella.[2,5] Early motion is advocated in isolated dislocation to attenuate pain, encourage quadriceps activity and maintain articular health. In patients with recurrent episodes of patella dislocation despite rehabilitation, a planned reconstructive surgery directed to their pathology is recommended.

However, severe effusion or haemarthrosis following patellar dislocation usually correlates with the severity of injury such as the presence of an osteochondral fracture. In patellar dislocation with concomitant osteochondral fracture, early surgical treatment in the form of MPFL repair, with fixation of the osteochondral fragment, is advised to restore the joint surface and to reduce the risk of further re-dislocation. The osteochondral lesions are thought to contribute to the development of post-traumatic patellofemoral joint osteoarthritis; therefore, early identification and referral for patellar dislocations, with fracture, benefits patients.

## Meniscus injury

Meniscus tears due to sports constitute 10% of all knee injuries, with the highest incidence of injuries occurring between ages 20 and 29 years old.[1] The incidence or prevalence in the older population is more difficult to ascertain due to the high prevalence of asymptomatic degenerative tears.

Meniscus tears are associated with development of post-traumatic osteoarthritis while knee osteoarthritis can itself lead to spontaneous meniscus tear. A population-based cross-sectional study using MRI scans showed that a meniscus tear is more common in men, the older age group and in those with an existing osteoarthritic knee but the radiological findings do not always correlate with functional symptoms.[6]

Swelling after a meniscus tear is of slower onset and less dramatic compared to ACL injury or acute patellar dislocation. It is more likely due to a twisting injury with the knee in a flexed position with combination of rotation or axial loading from a fall directly onto the knee. It can be associated with concomitant ligamentous injury, for example the triad of ACL, MCL and medial or lateral meniscus injuries. In an isolated meniscus tear, weight bearing is more likely immediately after injury although painful locked knee is a complication characteristically caused by bucket-handle tear, which demands urgent attention.

Suspected meniscus tear in patients older than 50 years old should be managed expectantly first. Physiotherapy should be commenced and may be supplemented by intra-articular injection of local anaesthetics and steroid for pain relief. If this fails to improve symptoms, the patient can be referred for orthopaedic review. Arthroscopic partial menisectomy is an option which can be discussed with patients, especially if they have mechanical symptoms like clicking, locking or 'giving way'. The benefits of arthroscopic surgery in the older age group are limited.[7]

In contrast, meniscus tears in young patients result from significant injury to the knee joint. MRI should be considered in younger and active patients with persistent knee pain, swelling, stiffness or lack of movement. A healthy or an intact meniscus protects against osteoarthritis. A knee joint with an intact meniscus (even after repair) gives better long-term outcomes compared to a knee after menisectomy. Repair of a meniscus tear should be considered in the younger population to allow a higher rate of achieving pre-injury sports activity. Patients undergoing meniscus repair should be counselled regarding the risk of reoperation due to failed repair and on the need for prolonged rehabilitation, especially avoiding deep flexion.

## Is this painful swollen knee septic arthritis?

Common causes of painful swollen knee in absence of injury include:

- Septic arthritis
- Gout/pseudogout
- Prepatellar bursitis
- Acute exacerbation of osteoarthritis
- Inflammatory arthritis

It can occasionally be difficult to differentiate between various causes of painful swollen knee.

---

### KEY POINTS – ACUTE KNEE INJURIES

- Knee swelling following a traumatic injury is secondary to bleeding in the joint and should be regarded as a serious injury until proven otherwise. Consider referring these patients urgently to a local acute knee injury clinic.
- Physical examination of an acutely injured knee is challenging but is an opportunity to determine severity of injury and prescribe appropriate management.
- A walking aid and knee immobiliser can be provided initially for a limited time frame while awaiting further assessments.
- If unsure of diagnosis on examination, consider specialist assessment to avoid missing significant injuries in patients with:
  - Haemarthrosis following injury
  - Significant bruising around knee
  - First episode of patella dislocation
  - Locked knee

---

Patients with septic arthritis usually have a combination of following features on presentation:

- Solitary joint pain
- Limited range of motion (ROM)
- Limping/inability to bear weight
- Fever

However, absence of these features would not always rule out infection in a joint. Neonates and the immunocompromised may not develop a febrile response. Even laboratory tests cannot completely exclude septic arthritis. A proportion of patients do not have a significantly raised erythrocyte sedimentation rate (ESR). Blood cultures are positive in only up to 50% of patients and joint aspirate cultures may be negative in 30% of aspirates. C-reactive protein (CRP), however, is a good negative predictor of septic arthritis. A CRP of <10 mg/L makes septic arthritis unlikely unless the patient is immunocompromised.

None of the tests in isolation has good sensitivity to detect septic arthritis but a combination of positive findings would help make a diagnosis. A combination of fever, inability to weight bear, ESR > 40 mm/h and white cell count (WCC) > 12 × 10⁹/L has sensitivity above 98%. Therefore, there needs to be a high clinical suspicion and these patients need to be referred urgently.

Patients with prepatellar bursitis may give a history of being involved in occupations involving kneeling. These patients usually are able to move their knee without any significant discomfort. There may be a history of pre-existing swelling/bursa in front of the patellar tendon. Swelling is located anterior to patellar tendon, and the knee itself is not swollen (Figure 7.6). The suprapatellar pouch of the knee extends about four finger-breadths proximal to patella. A large amount of fluid inside the knee joint leads to swelling proximal to the patella. Swelling from the prepatellar bursa is located anterior or inferior to the patella (Figure 7.7).

Patients with gout/pseudogout may have a pre-existing history of these conditions. Once the knee is swollen, it can be difficult to differentiate these from septic arthritis. Only way to differentiate would be to look for crystals on knee aspirate specimens.

Occasionally, patients with a known history of osteoarthritis or inflammatory arthritis can present with painful swollen knees with difficulty bearing weight on the affected limb. These patients are generally well and x-rays would help make a diagnosis. However, infection may coexist in arthritic joints. Blood tests and knee aspirate analysis are required to differentiate from infection.

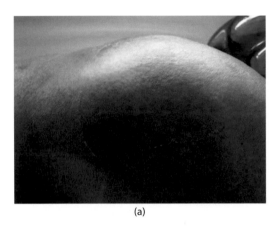

(a)

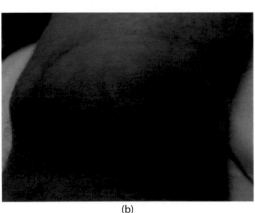

(b)

Figure 7.6 (a) Painful red diffuse swelling suggestive of septic arthritis. (b) Prepatellar bursitis: swelling localised to infrapatellar region with empty parapatellar and suprapatellar areas.

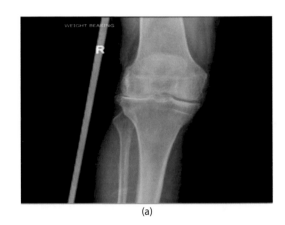

(a)

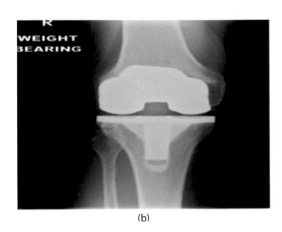

(b)

Figure 7.7 (a) Plain x-rays showing signs of osteoarthritis with loss of joint space. (b) Postoperative x-ray showing knee replacement.

## Red flag conditions: Malignancy

Knee pain can be rarely due to underlying malignancy. In adolescent and young adults, it is a site for primary bone sarcomas. An incidental history of injury may distract from an underlying diagnosis. The presence of rest pain in these patients can be a worrying feature. These patients should always have a plain x-rays and consider an MRI scan if there are any concerns on x-rays.

## Chronic knee conditions

## Osteoarthritis

Osteoarthritis of the knee joint is a common disabling condition in older patients; however, young to middle-aged patients are not immune to getting osteoarthritis symptoms.

## When do I refer patients with osteoarthritis for surgical management?

The National Institute for Health and Care Excellence (NICE) has provided guidance on management of chronic arthritis affecting knee joints. A holistic approach assessing patient's general health, socio-economic circumstances and effect on daily activities is recommended. As a first line of treatment, NICE recommends topical anti-inflammatory gel with oral paracetamol. If oral non-steroidal anti-inflammatory drugs (NSAIDs) or COX-2 inhibitor is prescribed, consider co-prescribing proton pump inhibitors. NICE does not recommend rubefacients or glucosamine/chondroitin products. All patients should be offered physiotherapy as a core treatment.

NICE recommends referring patients with osteoarthritis for surgery, if core treatments have failed and patients' symptoms have significant impact on their quality of life. NICE does not recommend use of any scoring tools or considering any patient specific factors like age, gender, smoking or obesity as a barrier for referral. It suggests that referral should be made before there is prolonged disability affecting patient function. If patients have significant limitation of activities of daily living and x-rays confirm significant osteoarthritis, patients should be referred to secondary care, after ruling out the hip as a source of pain.[8]

## Obese patients

It is a challenge to deliver the best outcome for obese patients. Various studies have suggested a higher complication rate for obese patients especially with oozing wounds and thromboembolic complications. However, if offered surgery, they improve equally well as compared to non-obese patients. However, there is not much evidence that these patients are more likely to lose weight following surgery due to improved mobility. For patients with BMI > 40 $kg/m^2$, a bariatric procedure prior to the knee replacement surgery may be advocated.

## Is there a role for arthroscopic surgery in knee osteoarthritis?

Arthroscopic surgery is usually not effective over the long term in the presence of established osteoarthritis.[7] Meniscal tears coexist with arthritis. It is difficult to discriminate meniscal symptoms from osteoarthritic symptoms. In older patients, arthroscopic surgery may occasionally be considered in patients without radiological arthritis, who present with acute effusion, well-localised joint line tenderness, catching or locking, following a specific mechanism of injury.

Patients should have a realistic understanding that the goal of arthroscopy is to diminish pain and improve function and not to cure their arthritis.

## Do I need to arrange an MRI scan for older patients with knee pain?

It is 'normal' to find 'abnormal' findings on an MRI scan in this age group. Twenty-four percent of patients with no arthritis would show a meniscal tear. Incidence of meniscal tears increases with the severity of OA (reaching up to 90% in severe OA). Asymptomatic patients would have a similar proportion of meniscal tears. There is not much of a role for MRI scans in patients older than 55 years.[6]

## What are the options for post-operative knee problems?

Common post-operative problems would include oozy wound, infection and thromboembolism. It is quite common for post-operative knees to look red and swollen. It can be very difficult to confirm infection. Starting oral antibiotics for suspected post-operative infections is not usually helpful. A short course of oral antibiotics may mask a real infection requiring urgent treatment. Most hospitals would give a contact number to patients to get in touch in case of a post-operative problem. Encourage patients to get in touch with the hospital or try to arrange it yourself, in case of a post-operative problem. It would be best for the patient to see an appropriate specialist to identify or refute a real post-operative problem.

## Injection technique

Patients appreciate their primary care physicians offering services like joint injections that traditionally require a referral to a specialist. Having these injections in a primary setting is a cost-effective option and avoids treatment delays. Injections help by providing short-term pain relief, and there is clinical evidence to support their use as part of a treatment package for osteoarthritis. Pain relief following injections may not be large or sustained over the long term but allows patients to commence their rehabilitation programme.

## What drugs should I use for injection?

Steroid injections are commonly used for intra-articular injections to the knee joint.

Commonly long-acting corticosteroid suspensions like methylprednisolone acetate (Depo-Medrol®) or triamcinolone acetonide (Kenalog® 40 mg/mL) formulations are used. It would be advisable to dilute steroid formulation in 10 mL of local anaesthetic to disperse steroid in large joint space. There are hyaluronic acid substitutes available in the market which are longer acting but are more expensive in comparison to steroid formulations.

## What are the contraindications to injecting a knee joint?

Absolute contraindications include local cellulitis, septic arthritis, acute fracture, artificial joint or history of allergy to injectable drugs. Relative contraindications include a known coagulopathy, current anticoagulation medication or uncontrolled diabetes. It is best to avoid steroid injections for quadriceps and patellar tendinopathy due to high risk of tendon rupture.

## What precautions should I take while injecting a knee joint?

Avoid injecting in subcutaneous tissues. Always aspirate before injection. The presence of joint fluid suggests the correct placement of needle tip, while blood on aspiration would need repositioning of the needle. It is reasonable to inject both knees at the same time, while taking care of maximum local anaesthetic dose. It is best to wait 3–4 months before considering repeating injections, with an aim of a maximum of three injections in a joint in 1 year. It may be reasonable to use injection therapy as a treatment choice in a medically unfit patient, following discussion with the patient. Don't use injections to delay surgical treatment in patients who may be best treated with a surgical procedure like knee replacement. There is a small risk of infection from intra-articular injections, which may complicate any future joint replacement surgery. Always take all aseptic precautions prior to injecting a joint.

## What are the possible complications of injection therapy?

There is a possibility of local anaesthetic toxicity or anaphylaxis response following any drug injection. Ask patients to wait for half an hour before going home. It is not uncommon to get a painful post-injection flare response. Warn patients about it and ask them to take some painkillers for the first few days. Injection into blood vessels can cause systemic effects. Infection in the joint is a rare but significant risk. Injection into subcutaneous tissues can cause skin hypopigmentation or atrophy.

## How do I inject a knee joint?

After explaining the procedure to the patient, get them to lie comfortably on a couch. There are different routes to inject a knee joint: mid-patellar, suprapatellar or infrapatellar (Figure 7.8).

The mid-patellar route is most accurate (Figure 7.9a and b). It can be done from either the lateral or medial side. It may be easier to inject from the medial side, as it is easier to evert the patella laterally. After prepping the skin, lift the medial edge of the patella and push the needle underneath the patella. There are no vital structures at risk but reposition if

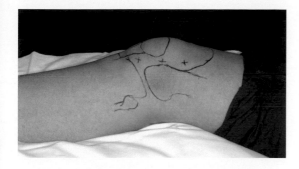

Figure 7.8 Side view of knee demonstrating extent of suprapatellar pouch and three possible portals for intra-articular injections (cross marks from top to bottom – suprapatellar, midpatellar, infrapatellar).

your hit bone or the articular surface. Aspirate and inject slowly.

The mid-patellar route may be difficult in patients with severe patella–femoral osteoarthritis due to osteophytes and fixed flexion deformity. In the presence of large effusion, it may be easier to put the needle in the suprapatellar pouch and inject after aspirating joint fluid (Figure 7.10a and b). In the absence of knee effusion, it may be easier to inject through the infrapatellar route in an arthritic knee. For this approach, ask the patient to keep the knee bent in about 90° flexion. Feel for the soft spot on either side of patella, above the tibia. Direct the needle towards the midline in front of the ACL and behind the fat pad (Figure 7.11a and b).

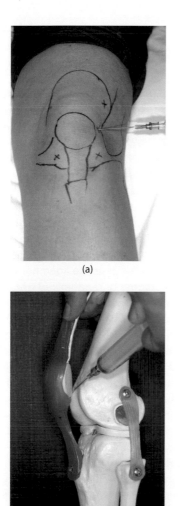

(a)

(b)

Figure 7.9 (a) and (b) Midpatellar approach to knee injection.

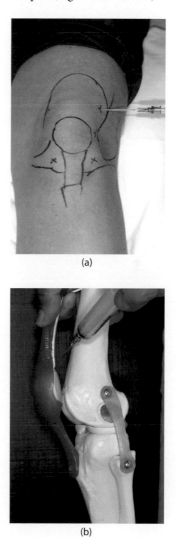

(a)

(b)

Figure 7.10 (a) and (b) Suprapatellar approach to knee injection.

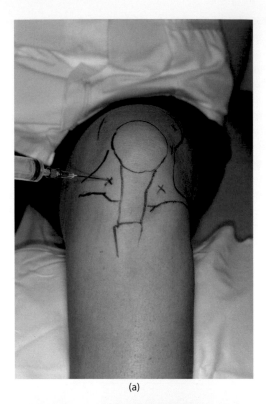

(a)

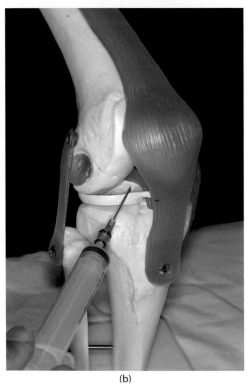

(b)

Figure 7.11 **(a)** and **(b)** Infrapatellar approach to knee injection.

## SUMMARY POINTS – CHRONIC KNEE PROBLEMS

- Chronic knee problems can be a source of significant morbidity.
- It is reasonable to give a trial of conservative treatment.
- Patients should be advised on lifestyle modifications and weight loss.
- Referral to secondary care should not be delayed if there is poor response to non-operative measures.

## References

1. Bollen S. Ligament injuries of the knee—Limping forward? *Br J Sports Med.* 1998;32(1):82–84.
2. Lee L, Khan M, Anand S. Acute soft tissue knee injuries. *InnovAiT: Education and Inspiration for General Practice.* 2014;7(7):428–436.
3. Voskanian N. ACL Injury prevention in female athletes: Review of the literature and practical considerations in implementing an ACL prevention program. *Curr Rev Musculoskelet Med.* 2013;6(2):158–163.
4. Frobell R, Roos H, Roos E, Roemer F, Ranstam J, Lohmander L. Treatment for acute anterior cruciate ligament tear: Five year outcome of randomised trial. *BMJ.* 2013;346(Jan 24):f232.
5. Sillanpää P, Mattila VM, Iivonen T, Visuri T, Pihlajamäki H. Incidence and risk factors of acute traumatic primary patellar dislocation. *Med Sci Sports Exerc.* 2008;40(4):606–611.
6. Englund M, Guermazi A, Gale D, Hunter D, Aliabadi P, Clancy M et al. Incidental meniscal findings on knee MRI in middle-aged and elderly persons. *N Engl J Med.* 2008;359(11):1108–1115.
7. Thorlund J, Juhl C, Roos E, Lohmander L. Arthroscopic surgery for degenerative knee: Systematic review and meta-analysis of benefits and harms. *BMJ.* 2015;350(Jun 16):h2747–h2747.
8. NICE. Nice.org.uk. 2016 [cited 3 August 2016]. https://www.nice.org.uk/guidance/cg177/evidence/full-guideline-191761309.

# 8

# Foot and ankle disorders

MANEESH BHATIA

## Introduction

Foot and ankle problems are quite common in the community. To put this in perspective, at any given time, 10%–15% of the population suffers from heel pain alone.

Unfortunately, due to a number of interlinked structures, it can be hard to diagnose and treat these problems. It would not be realistic to expect from a general practitioner (GP) detailed knowledge regarding the anatomy and pathology of all these structures. The objective of this chapter is to help the GP understand the management of common foot and ankle problems seen in primary care.

Fortunately, in most cases, there is a well-localised area of pain and tenderness. In my experience, eliciting localised tenderness is a very useful diagnostic tool. I have divided the foot and ankle into different zones to highlight the most common pathologies involving these zones (Figure 8.1).

## Achilles rupture

### Introduction

Although Achilles ruptures are not commonly seen in primary care, a missed diagnosis has significant implications.

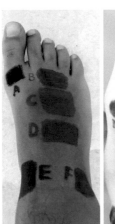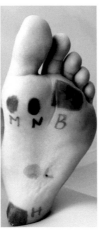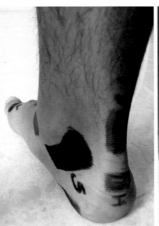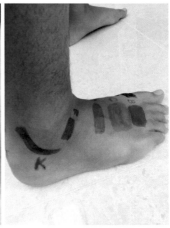

Figure 8.1 Zones of foot and ankle highlighting most common pathologies associated with these areas. **(a)** Arthritis of first metatarsophalangeal (MTP) joint. **(b)** Morton's neuroma, synovitis of MTP joint (usually second). **(c)** Stress fracture (or bone marrow oedema) of metatarsal (sudden history of pain accompanied with marked swelling is usually due to a stress fracture or bone marrow oedema which is seen in magnetic resonance imaging [MRI] scan). **(d)** Arthritis of tarso metatarsal joints (usually second and third). **(e)** Ankle arthritis or impingement ankle (anteromedial). **(f)** Ankle arthritis or impingement ankle (anterolateral) or sinus tarsi syndrome. **(g)** Tibialis posterior tendon problem. **(h)** Plantar fasciitis. **(i)** Insertional Achilles tendon problems. **(j)** Non-insertional Achilles tendon problems. **(k)** Peroneal tendon problems. **(l)** Pain could be due to plantar fasciitis, swelling in this area is usually due to plantar fibroma. **(m)** Medial sesamoid inflammation. **(n)** Lateral sesamoid inflammation.

## What causes Achilles rupture?

The factors leading to rupture of achilles can be divided into two categories:

1. *Intrinsic factors:* This tendon bears high loads. It is estimated that up to 10 times body weight goes across this tendon when running. In addition, it spans three joints (knee, ankle and subtalar joints). There is a zone of relative avascularity, 2–6 cm proximal to its insertion. Most of the Achilles tendon ruptures occur in this region.
2. *Extrinsic factors:* These include mechanical factors (overpronation), hyperthermia (sudden exposure to increased temperatures, the classical example being lack of warm-up prior to running or sports), medication (steroids and flouroquinolones) and iatrogenic (steroid injection) (Figure 8.2).

## What is the incidence of Achilles ruptures?

At Leicester Royal Infirmary, we treat about 90–100 patients with Achilles rupture every year (catchment population about 1.1 million). It is much more commonly seen in males with the male/female ratio being 4.2:1, and the average age being 47 years in our experience.

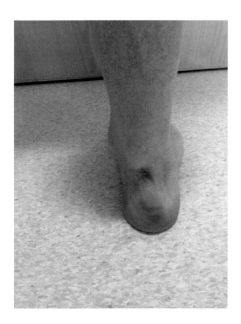

Figure 8.2 Achilles rupture following steroid injection.

## Why is this injury missed?

Unfortunately, the diagnosis of Achilles rupture could be delayed or missed leading to litigation. There are several reasons for a missed diagnosis. The initial pain following Achilles rupture settles within the first few days after injury. The patient might not therefore present immediately. Sometimes, the patient self-diagnoses this as an ankle sprain. I have seen cases where the initial injury happened when the patient was abroad and presented after some time to his or her GP. Diagnosing this injury after a while can be challenging due to swelling and hematoma, which can mask the gap. In my view, the most common reason of missing this injury is due to the fact that the diagnosis of Achilles rupture has not crossed the mind of the examiner. Sometimes, the diagnosis might have been considered, but as the patient was able to move foot up and down, the diagnosis of ruptured Achilles was excluded. Remember that the patient would be able to plantar flex the foot in the presence of Achilles rupture as the other plantar flexors (tibialis posterior, flexor digitorum and flexor hallucis longus [FHL]) are functioning.

## How to diagnose Achilles rupture

It is important to consider the diagnosis of Achilles rupture when examining a patient with a calf or ankle injury. Alarm bells should ring regarding possible Achilles rupture if a patient tells you that 'It felt as if somebody kicked me in the calf, however when I turned back there was nobody'.

**Examination:** A gap is palpable at the site of rupture (usually about 4 cm proximal to the insertion of Achilles). However, this becomes difficult with a delayed presentation. The most reliable clinical test is the *calf squeeze test* (also known as the *Simmonds or Thompson test*). This test has very high sensitivity and specificity. The second test to aid the diagnosis is the *single heel raise test*. **If there is plantar flexion of the foot on calf squeeze and the patient is able to perform a single heel raise, Achilles rupture is highly unlikely** (Figure 8.3). One other clinical finding seen in cases of an old Achilles rupture is excessive dorsiflexion of the ankle on the ruptured side.

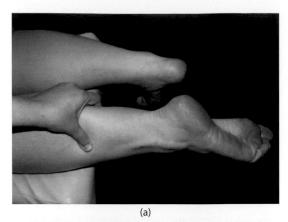

(a)

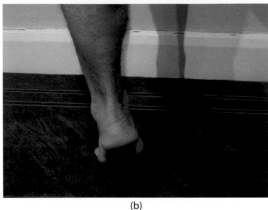

(b)

Figure 8.3 Clinical tests showing intact Achilles tendon: **(a)** calf squeeze test and **(b)** single heel raise test.

## What are the treatment options for Achilles rupture?

Historically, this injury was treated by either open surgery or non-surgically in a plaster cast. Those who would favour surgery would quote a high re-rupture rate (up to 13%) with the non-surgical treatment. On the other hand, the incidence of infection/wound-healing complications following open surgical repair has been reported to be about 5%.

In the last few years, non-surgical, weight-bearing functional mobilisation has gained momentum. There are many studies which have shown good outcomes and low re-rupture rate with this treatment.[1] We have been treating most of these injuries with a VACOped boot since 2009 and in our experience, the re-rupture rate of Achilles tendon with non-surgical, weight-bearing functional mobilisation (8/52) is 2%–3% (Figure 8.4).

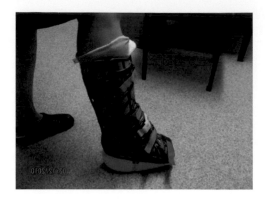

Figure 8.4 VACOped boot for treatment of Achilles rupture.

A case for surgery can be made for high-demand patients who are engaged in sporting activities. Minimum invasive repair avoids the risks of open surgery and results in quicker rehabilitation.

**Take home message:** Consider the diagnosis of Achilles rupture in lower leg, calf or ankle injuries. *'It felt that somebody kicked me in the calf'* should ring an alarm bell. The calf squeeze and single heel raise tests are the most important clinical diagnostic tests.

## Achilles tendinopathy

### Introduction

Traditionally, Achilles tendon pain has been referred to as Achilles tendonitis. However, studies have shown absence of inflammatory mediators in tendon biopsies of chronic Achilles tendinosis. Interestingly, the concentrations of glutamate, which is a potent mediator of pain, have been found in higher concentrations in these cases.[2] The term Achilles tendonitis has therefore been replaced by Achilles tendinosis (pathological) or Achilles tendinopathy (clinical).

### What are the two types of Achilles tendinopathy?

The classification is based on the location of swelling and tenderness:

1. *Mid-substance (non-insertional) tendinopathy:* The swelling is seen about 5–6 cm proximal to the insertion of the Achilles tendon (Figure 8.5).

Although it is frequently seen in runners, it can affect the sedentary population as well.

2. *Insertional tendinopathy*: The tenderness and swelling is localised at the insertion of Achilles tendon. The enlarged posterolateral part of the calcaneum is known as **'Haglund's process or deformity'**. One of the other synonyms of this condition is **'pump bump'** (Figure 8.6).

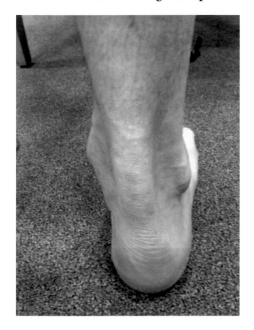

Figure 8.5 Midsubstance (non-insertional) Achilles tendinopathy.

## What is the clinical presentation?

The presenting symptoms are pain, swelling and stiffness. In the initial stages, there is 'first-step pain and stiffness'. Pain is triggered with activities and relieved by rest. In chronic cases, pain becomes constant.

## What is the management of Achilles tendinopathy?

In the vast majority of patients, the symptoms settle within 2–4 weeks not requiring any further treatment. If pain continues after 4 weeks, *eccentric stretching* exercises of the Achilles tendon (*heel drop*) should be tried. The patient should be warned that initially these exercises could lead to aggravation of pain. He or she should therefore be advised to take analgesics and non-steroidal anti-inflammatory drugs (NSAIDs) on a regular basis, to be able to continue eccentric stretching for at least 6 weeks. If this does not result in improvement, other measures can be tried which include:

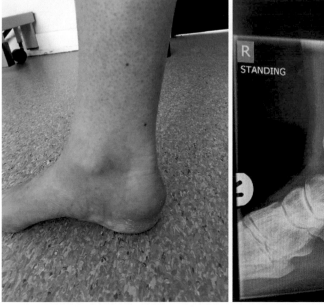
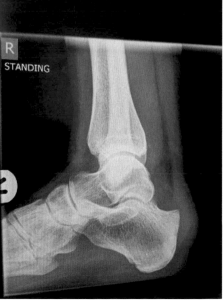

Figure 8.6 Insertional Achilles tendinopathy and Haglund's deformity.

**Shock wave therapy (SWT):** This treatment modality has become quite popular recently. It is a non-invasive intervention and can be used for both non-insertional and insertional Achilles tendinopathy. It is an outpatient procedure and involves application of SWT at the area of tenderness. Each treatment cycle takes about 5 minutes. It is done at a weekly interval and usually about 3–6 sessions are recommended. It is a low-risk procedure. It acts by stimulating the body's healing response. The success rate of this treatment in my experience is 70%.

**Ultrasound-guided dry needling and high-volume saline infiltration:** This is an ultrasound-guided procedure performed by the radiologist and involves needling of the Achilles tendon along with infiltration of a high volume of saline (30–50 mL). The success rate of this procedure in our experience is 60%.

**Ultrasound-guided steroid injection:** This procedure is indicated sometimes for insertional tendinopathy specially for *retrocalcaneal bursitis*. I would like to emphasise that (1) this should not be performed for non-insertional tendinopathy and (2) blind steroid injections for Achilles tendinopathy should not be performed in primary care because of the risk of rupture of Achilles.

## Role of surgery

**Non-insertional tendinopathy:** The overlying layer (paratenon) is stripped from the underlying tendon. Achilles tendon debridement and repair are performed. In severe tendinopathy, Achilles tendon reconstruction using FHL tendon transfer might be required.

**Insertional tendinopathy:** Heel bone prominence (Haglund's process) and the calcified/degenerate part of Achilles tendon are excised. The Achilles tendon is reattached to the calcaneum with the help of bone anchor sutures.

If there is undue tightness of gastrocnemius muscle then some surgeons believe that releasing the tight fascia of this muscle can be beneficial. Postoperatively, a plaster/boot is applied for 2–6 weeks depending on the surgery. This is followed by physiotherapy for about 6 weeks. The success rate of surgery is 80%–90%.

**Take home message:** Do not inject an Achilles tendon with steroids as this can lead to rupture. Non-surgical treatment is successful for the majority. Surgical treatment can be considered if symptoms do not improve with conventional treatment.

## Ankle arthritis

## What causes it?

In the vast majority of patients with ankle arthritis, there is a history of previous injury either in the form of a sprain or fracture of the ankle. The other common cause is inflammatory arthritis.

## How to diagnose it

The presenting complains are pain, swelling and stiffness around the ankle joint. Tenderness can be elicited on anteromedial and anterolateral aspects of the ankle. In early arthritis, the movements of the ankle joint are usually preserved. There might be varus or valgus deformity of the hindfoot in severe cases. X-rays are helpful to confirm the diagnosis.

## What is the treatment?

1. The non-invasive treatment measures include oral and topical anti-inflammatories, use of an ankle brace or lace-up boots, activity modification, weight loss and stick support in the opposite hand.
2. Steroid injection can be considered in early arthritis. It can be done by an anteromedial (Figure 8.7) or anterolateral approach.
3. The efficacy of hyaluronic acid in treating ankle arthritis is not proven.
4. *Arthroscopic ankle debridement:* Arthroscopic surgery has a role in early arthritis. It is not effective in severe arthritis.
5. *Distal tibial (supramalleolar) osteotomy:* It is an option to be considered for the treatment of moderate arthritis in young patients. It is indicated if the arthritis is confined to one-half (medial or lateral) of the ankle joint.
6. *Ankle fusion also known as ankle arthrodesis:* Ankle arthrodesis is usually performed arthroscopically these days. This operation is indicated for young patients with high functional demands (Figure 8.8).

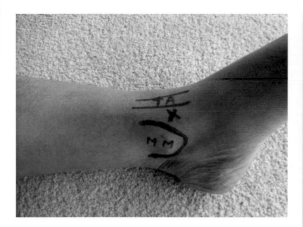

Figure 8.7 Anteromedial approach for ankle injection.

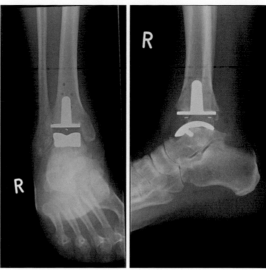

Figure 8.9 Ankle replacement.

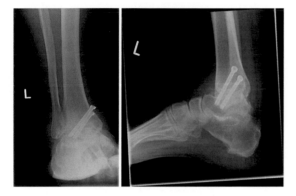

Figure 8.8 Arthroscopic ankle fusion.

7. Ankle replacement also known as ankle arthroplasty (Figure 8.9): Ankle arthroplasty has become popular in the last few years.[3] It helps in preserving movements of the ankle thereby relieving pressure on neighbouring joints as compared to ankle arthrodesis. The modern arthroplasty implants have resulted in improved longitivity and better results. The survivorship of one make of ankle replacements (Hintegra) has been reported to be 84% at 10 years for a group of 684 patients.[4] An ideal candidate for ankle replacement is a patient with low functional demand usually greater than 65 years. It can be considered for younger patients with rheumatoid arthritis. The presence of a significant deformity is a contraindication for ankle replacement.

**Take home message:** Ankle arthritis is usually posttraumatic. Ankle fusion is the gold standard treatment for end-stage arthritis. Though ankle replacement is not as successful as hip and knee replacement, the results are improving and can lead to a good outcome in carefully selected patients.

# Bunion (hallux valgus)

## Introduction

The term bunion is derived from the Latin word 'bunio' which means turnip. A bunion, therefore, refers to an enlargement typically on the medial aspect of the great toe. Hallux valgus on the other hand describes the deformity normally associated with a bunion (hallux = great toe; valgus = outward deviation).

The most common cause of hallux valgus is genetic. Shoes causing increased pressure on fore-foot (pointed shoes with narrow toe box along with high heels) can accelerate progression of the deformity, especially in genetically predisposed patients. The other contributory factor is *pes planovalgus (flatfeet)*. Hallux valgus is also associated with arthritis, especially rheumatoid arthritis.

## What is the clinical presentation?

The presentation could be due to pain localised around the bunion. On the other hand, in quite a few cases, the bunion might not be painful, but the hallux valgus deformity could lead to secondary problems such as pain around the second toe metatarsophalangeal (MTP) joint due to synovitis, claw toe or hammer toe deformity affecting lesser toes, Morton's neuroma and metatarsalgia. I have seen stress fractures of lesser metatarsals due to increased pressure as a result of an inefficient first ray.

## What is the treatment?

Insoles and orthotics have no major role in the treatment of bunions. Having said that, a medial arch support can help bunions in the presence of flatfeet. For patients who are unfit for surgery, custom-made wide fitting shoes can be useful.

**Surgical treatment:** The primary problem leading to hallux valgus is the underlying deformity of the first metatarsal and proximal phalanx bones. Therefore, simply removing the bunion (bunionectomy) leads to almost 100% recurrence. The surgical treatment for hallux valgus correction involves metatarsal and phalangeal osteotomies in addition to bunionectomy and soft tissue release (Figure 8.10).

## What is the recovery following surgery?

The foot needs to be protected in a heel wedge shoe for a minimum period of 6 weeks post-surgery. The patient can start weight bearing almost immediately after the operation in this shoe. It can take 7–8 weeks to drive a manual transmission car after this surgery. Overall, recovery can take 3–4 months. Patients should be warned that there could be some swelling of the foot after any foot surgery for up to 12 months (Figure 8.11).

**Take home message:** Non-surgical measures are not effective for hallux valgus treatment. An asymptomatic bunion with significant hallux valgus can cause problems related to lesser toes.

## Arthritis of great toe (hallux rigidus)

### Introduction

This is the most common site of arthritis in the foot. The incidence is 2% over the age of 50 years.

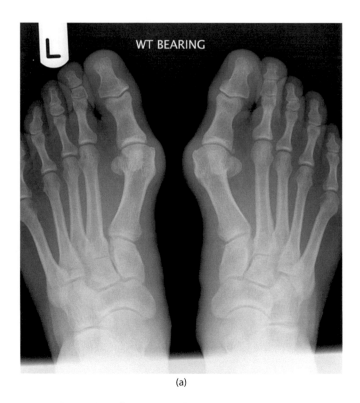
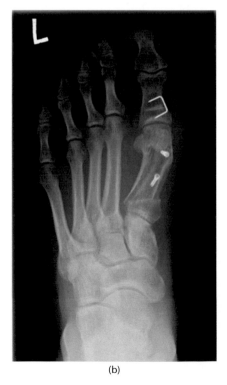

(a)  (b)

Figure 8.10 **(a)** Hallux valgus deformity and **(b)** hallux valgus correction (scarf and akin osteotomies).

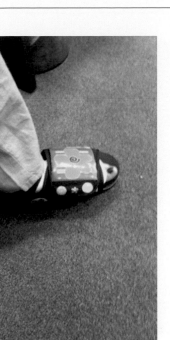

Figure 8.11 DARCO shoe for weight-bearing mobilisation after first ray surgery.

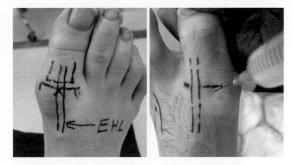

Figure 8.12 Steroid injection for hallux rigidus.

## What is the cause?

The most common cause is primary arthritis. The other causes include trauma, hallux valgus, rheumatoid arthritis and gout.

## What is the presentation?

The most common presenting features are pain, swelling and stiffness. It can be sometimes confused with gout. Gout usually has an acute onset with diffused soft tissue swelling and erythema around the big toe. Hallux rigidus, on the other hand, has an insidious onset with localised swelling on the dorsum of the MTP joint. In early stages, the extremes of movements are painful. As the arthritis progresses, the range of movements becomes limited. This is the reason for using terms such as hallux rigidus or limitus for this condition. X-rays are required for the confirmation of clinical diagnosis.

## What is the treatment?

***Non-surgical treatment:*** Activity and shoe wear modification along with NSAIDs can be tried in the treatment of early arthritis. A stiff soled shoe or a shoe with a rocker sole reduces movements of first MTP joint and midfoot, thereby improving pain.

*Steroid injection*: A steroid injection can be tried in early arthritis (Figure 8.12).

**Surgery**

*Cheilectomy*: For patients with pain only on terminal movements and a palpable dorsal bone spur (osteophyte), the cheilectomy procedure is indicated. This is usually the case in mild/moderate arthritis.

For the late stage of arthritis, *fusion/arthrodesis* is the gold standard surgery. There is a good success rate in the order of 90% following MTP joint fusion (Figure 8.13).

## What is new in the treatment of the arthritis of the first MTP joint?

Although joint fusion surgery (arthrodesis) is a very good operation for pain relief, many patients especially females do not like the idea of joint fusion surgery as this leads to a stiff joint limiting the choice of shoe wear. An alternative treatment is using a synthetic cartilage implant called *Cartiva*. Cartiva is a synthetic cartilage plug (polyvinyl alcohol hydrogel), which is composed of material with properties similar to those of native cartilage. It is softer than metal and has similar strength as that of human cartilage. It works as a spacer in the joint thereby separating the joint surfaces and therefore improves the pain and preserves movement. There has been a multination, multicentre study comparing Cartiva with joint fusion surgery. At 2-year follow-up, there is no difference in

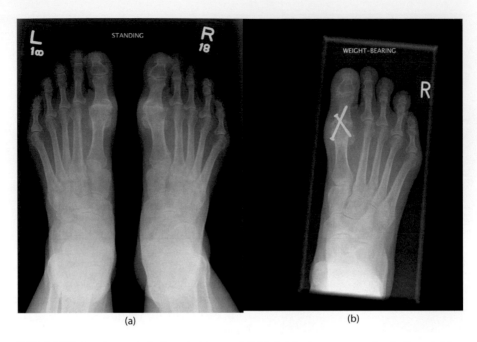

Figure 8.13 **(a)** Bilateral severe hallux rigidus and **(b)** joint fusion surgery for hallux rigidus.

outcome between the two procedures. The risk of failure of Cartiva at 2 years is 10%.[5]

**Take home message:** Steroid injections are quite effective for early arthritis of the big toe. If the symptoms are related to pain on push off/forced dorsiflexion, cheilectomy can be helpful. First MTP joint fusion is a good treatment for end-stage arthritis. The early results of joint sparing surgery (Cartiva, artificial cartilage plug) are encouraging.

## Plantar fasciitis

### Introduction

This condition is the most common cause of heel pain in adults. It is estimated that up to 15% cases of foot pain can be attributed to this condition. Plantar fasciitis is considered a self-limited condition. Symptoms resolve in the majority (70%) of cases within 3 months.

### What is the pathology?

Repeated mechanical overload produces micro tears within the plantar fascia, leading to an inflammatory response. The normal healing response is prevented by chronic overuse and repeated heel strikes.

The most common site of involvement is the medial band of plantar fascia at the calcaneal origin.

### Who is at risk?

The most important risk factors are as follows:

1. Reduced ankle dorsiflexion or tightness of Achilles
2. Increased body mass index (BMI)
3. Runners
4. Individuals who stand a lot (this is the reason for the old acronym, *Policeman's heel*)

### What is the clinical picture?

The classical clinical picture of plantar fasciitis is the so-called *'first-step pain'*. This sharp, stabbing pain is usually localised to the plantar medial aspect of the heel and occurs first thing in the morning or after sitting for a long period. This pain and stiffness improves after weight bearing. Gradually however, this can change to a constant pain or ache. The tenderness can most commonly be elicited at the medial aspect of the calcaneum. Sometimes, there is localised tenderness around the central band of plantar fascia. The lateral aspect of the heel is rarely involved.

In most cases, there is associated Achilles and/or hamstring tightness as well. If the dorsiflexion of ankle improves with knee flexion, this represents isolated tightness of gastrocnemius muscle.

## What is the treatment?

1. *Stretching of plantar fascia and Achilles tendon:* This simple and inexpensive treatment should be the first line of treatment. Plantar fascia-specific stretching (dorsiflexion of big toe) can result in early improvement in pain.
2. *Night splints:* During sleep, the foot is plantar flexed. This causes contracture of the Achilles and plantar fascia and is responsible for first-step pain. Night splints keep the foot in dorsiflexion thereby preventing the contracture of the Achilles and plantar fascia. There is good evidence to support the use of a night splint. They can be bought online.
3. *Orthoses:* Although there is some benefit from the use of heel cups and heel pads, the evidence is not as good as that for stretching and night splints. Firm foam or semirigid plastic is superior to soft foam.
4. *Non-steroid anti-inflammatory agents:* Review of literature suggests that this provides short-term relief, and the effect is usually limited to about a month.
5. *Corticosteroid injections:* Although steroid injections can provide short-term relief there is a significant risk of recurrence. Repeated, multiple injections given in the central heel pad can lead to fat pad atrophy and rupture/tear of the plantar fascia. A single injection applied medially at the bone fascia interface should be combined with stretching or use of a night splint.
6. *Platelet rich plasma (PRP) or autologous blood injections:* These injections have gained increasing popularity to treat tendinopathies and fasciopathies. However, the current evidence in literature regarding the efficacy of these injections is mixed.[6]
7. *Extra corporeal SWT (ESWT):* This treatment modality has evolved in the last 10 years. It is supposed to act by increase in growth factors locally thereby stimulating the healing/repair process. This treatment is administered in an outpatient setting every week for 3–6 weeks. The advantage of this treatment is that there are no significant adverse effects. I have audited and published my results for ESWT which are in line with current literature. In our audit, 85% cases have reported improvement in their symptoms.
8. *Surgery:*
   a. *Direct release of plantar fascia:* This treatment has become almost obsolete due to risk of complications as high as 50%.
   b. *Indirect release:* This surgical treatment has evolved in the last few years and is favoured by surgeons as it is a safer surgical treatment as compared to direct release of the plantar fascia. It involves release of the fascia overlying the medial head of the gastrocnemius in the proximal calf. There is good evidence to support the role of this surgery for chronic plantar fasciitis which has not responded to conventional treatment.

**Take home message:** There is a good chance that symptoms of plantar fasciitis will improve in the first 3 months. Stretching exercises for the plantar fascia, Achilles and hamstrings should be tried before an invasive intervention. Repeated multiple steroid injections in the central heel pad should be avoided. SWT is safe and can be effective. For reluctant cases, surgery in the form of medial gastrocnemius release can be attempted.

# Flatfoot (pes planus) in adults

## What is flatfoot?

Absence or loss of medial arch of the foot is defined as flatfoot.

## What are the types of flatfoot in adults?

There are two types of flatfoot in adults:

1. *Physiological:* This is bilateral and symmetrical. The flatfoot deformity is flexible. This is usually asymptomatic and does not require surgical treatment.
2. *Pathological:* This is usually unilateral or bilateral and asymmetrical. The deformity is rigid. The patients are symptomatic. The deformity

is progressive. This group of patients should be diagnosed and treated soon as delay in management affects the treatment and prognosis.

There are two simple clinical tests to differentiate between these two conditions:

1. *Heel raise test:* When the patient stands on the toes, the heels go into varus (face each other) and the fallen arch is formed in a patient with flexible flatfeet (Figure 8.14).
2. *Jack's test:* The involved foot is rested on a flat surface. The great toe is passively dorsiflexed (lifted off the ground). In flexible deformity, the arch reforms (Figure 8.15).

## What are the causes of pathological flatfoot?

The most common cause for this condition in adults is *tibialis posterior dysfunction.* The other causes are tarsal coalition (congenital condition where bones in the midfoot and hindfoot are abnormally joined together), and posttraumatic and rheumatoid arthritis.

## What is tibialis posterior tendon dysfunction?

The tibialis posterior tendon is one of the most important tendons in the foot. It has two functions:

(a) it supports the arch of the foot and (b) it is the strongest invertor of the foot and ankle. Problems with this tendon lead to a flattened arch (pes planus or flatfoot) and a progressive valgus deformity. Tibialis posterior dysfunction is common in middle-aged females. The other predisposing factors for problems with this disorder include obesity, diabetes, hypertension, preexisting pes planus, steroid use and trauma.

## What are the clinical features of tibialis posterior tendon dysfunction?

The most common presentation is acute onset of pain and swelling on the medial aspect of the ankle behind and distal to medial malleolus. This is followed by progressive planovalgus deformity (loss of arch and valgus of the heel). The deformity is best appreciated from behind and is described as the '*too many toes sign*'. A simple clinical test is inability to perform a single heel raise (Figure 8.16).

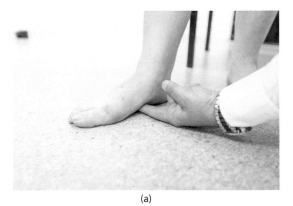

(a)

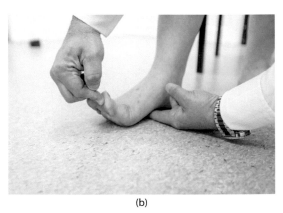

(b)

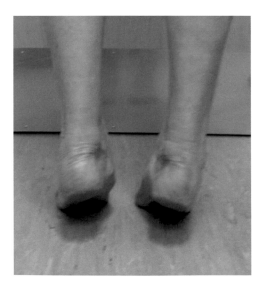

Figure 8.14 Heel raise test showing flexible flatfeet.

Figure 8.15 **(a)** and **(b)** Jack's test showing restoration of medial arch on dorsiflexion of big toe for flexible pes planus.

## What are the stages of tibialis posterior dysfunction?

As this is a progressive condition, it has been classified into four stages:

*Stage I:* Acute stage of medial pain and swelling. This is due to tenosynovitis and the tendon is intact. There is no deformity, and the patient can perform a single heel raise.

*Stage II:* Tendon is torn and is weak. The deformity is correctible. On bilateral heel raise, the valgus deformity corrects. The patient cannot perform a single heel raise.

*Stage III:* There is a fixed valgus deformity, which does not correct on bilateral heel raise test. The patient cannot perform a single heel raise.

*Stage IV:* In addition to the above, this is associated with radiographic changes of arthritis.

## What is the treatment of tibialis posterior dysfunction?

The treatment is dependent on the stage of the disease.

*Stage I:* Immobilisation in plaster cast for 6 weeks followed by physiotherapy.

*Stages II and III:* Tibialis posterior reconstruction surgery. This involves tendon transfer and medial displacement calcaneal osteotomy. The patient is in plaster for 6 weeks followed by physiotherapy. It takes 3–6 months to recover from this operation. The success rate is in the order of 80%–90%.

*Stage IV:* This involves triple fusion. The patient is in plaster for 3 months followed by physiotherapy. It takes 6–12 months to recover and leads to stiffness of hindfoot joints.

**Take home message:** The most important cause of pathological flatfoot in adults is tibialis posterior dysfunction. It is important to diagnose and treat this early as delay can lead to fixed deformity with arthritis.

## Cavovarus deformity

### What does cavovarus deformity mean?

Cavus represents a high arch. This is best appreciated from side. Varus deformity means that the hind feet rather than being in a neutral position are medially inclined (heels facing each other). Varus is best appreciated from behind (Figure 8.17).

### What are the causes of cavovarus deformity?

Although in quite a few cases there is no known cause (idiopathic), this deformity can be associated with a neurological cause such as Charcot–Marie–Tooth disease, cerebral palsy, spinal problems or polio. On the other hand, a varus deformity on its own can be due to significant ankle arthritis (usually posttraumatic commonly resulting from an old severe lateral ligament or peroneal tendon injury).

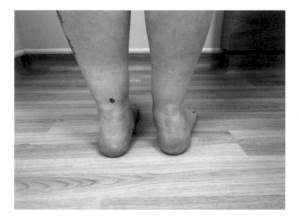

Figure 8.16 Too many toes sign on right side.

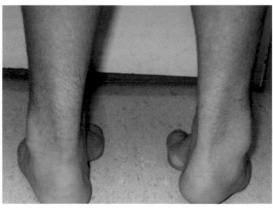

Figure 8.17 Bilateral cavovarus deformity.

## What is the treatment?

In early stages, orthotics can be tried for a flexible deformity. However, this being a progressive deformity, a surgical intervention is indicated in most cases. In early stages, tendon transfers and osteotomies can be considered. In cases of fixed deformity, joint fusion surgery is required.

**Take home message:** Consider a neurological cause when examining a cavovarus deformity. This usually requires specialist surgical intervention and therefore should be referred to secondary care.

## Morton's neuroma

### What is Morton's neuroma?

Morton's neuroma is one of the most frequent causes of localised forefoot pain. The pain is due to thickened tissues surrounding interdigital nerve (perineural fibrosis). It is seen in the third and/or second intermetatarsal space. It is commonly seen in runners. The other causes include hallux valgus deformity, ill-fitting shoes, inflammatory arthritis, trauma and idiopathic. Morton's neuroma is more commonly seen in females.

### What is the clinical presentation?

The pain is localised on the under surface (plantar aspect) of the forefoot. Sometimes, this radiates to the second or third toes. Patients can report numbness/altered sensation of the tip of one or more toes. The pain is on weight bearing and there is usually no rest pain.

Removing the shoe might improve the pain in the early stage. However, in chronic cases, the pain becomes constant. Some patients may also describe as if they feel a pebble in the shoe when walking.

## How to diagnose Morton's neuroma

The diagnosis is essentially clinical. The history is often suggestive of the diagnosis. The simplest and sensitive clinical test is the *'thumb index finger squeeze test'* (Figure 8.18).

*Mulder's click test* is elicited by dorsiflexion of the foot and squeezing the toes. This test can miss small neuromas.

## What is the treatment?

Initial treatment is usually non-surgical including activity and footwear modification, anti-inflammatory medication and cortisone injection (Figure 8.19).

**Surgical treatment:** Surgery is considered when the conservative treatment is not helpful. It involves excision of the interdigital nerve along with the neuroma (Figure 8.20).

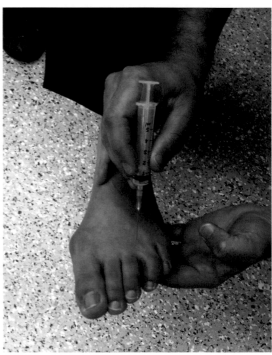

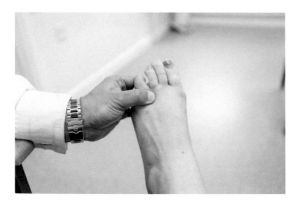

Figure 8.18 Thumb index finger squeeze test to elicit tenderness for clinical diagnosis of Morton's neuroma.

Figure 8.19 Steroid injection for Morton's neuroma.

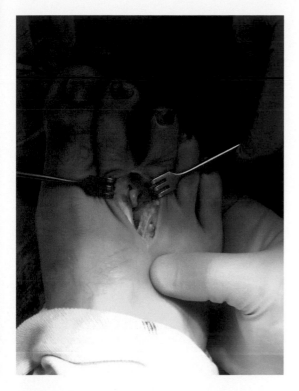

Figure 8.20 Intraoperative picture of Morton's neuroma.

**Take home message:** Morton's neuroma is the most common cause of pain between lesser toes. It can be caused by repeated impact secondary to running or high heels, overcrowding usually due to hallux valgus or trauma. Clinical diagnosis is fairly accurate. When in doubt, an ultrasound scan can be useful. Activity and shoe modification is useful in the early stages. Steroid injection is a good adjunct for treatment. Surgery can be performed for reluctant cases; however, the recurrence rate is as high as 20%.

## Ankle sprains

### Introduction

This is the most common sporting injury. However, it can occur in the non-sporting population as well during day-to-day activities.

### What is the clinical presentation?

The vast majority of cases are following an inversion injury. The presentation is variable depending on the severity of the injury. The time taken for the swelling, amount of swelling and bruising and ability to bear weight are important clues with regard to severity of the sprain. In addition, in case of a severe ankle sprain, the patient might report an audible loud noise mimicking fracture.

### Which ligaments are involved in common ankle sprains?

The most commonly seen is inversion injury, which involves the lateral ligament complex that comprises the anterior talofibular ligament (ATFL) and the calcaneofibular ligament (CFL).

### What is the classification of ankle sprains?

*Grade I:* The ligament is stretched. There is mild swelling and bruising.
*Grade II:* There is partial tear of the ligaments. Gross instability is not a feature.
*Grade III:* There is complete tear of the ligaments. In the acute stage, the patient is unable to bear weight. There is marked instability with a positive anterior drawer test.

### What is the prognosis of ankle sprains?

Patients with mild (Grade I) ankle sprains improve within a couple of weeks. Most patients with a Grade II injury get better by about 6–12 weeks after injury. However, up to 40% of patients suffering from a Grade III sprain do not improve and suffer from pain and/or instability.

### What is the treatment of acute ankle sprains?

Treatment of the acute sprain includes conventional measures (rest, ice or cold packs, compression, elevation, NSAIDs). If symptoms do not settle in 3 months, a referral to secondary care is advised.

### What are the indications for surgery?

There are two indications for surgery:

1. *Pain:* This is seen in about 20%–40% patients with Grade III sprains. This is due to soft tissue

impingement. Arthroscopic surgery is quite effective to deal with this.

2. *Instability:* This is seen in up to one-third of patients with Grade III sprains. An anatomic ligament reconstruction (Brostrom repair) has been reported as the gold standard of surgical treatment with good functional outcome in 90% patients.

**Take home message:** Ninety-five percent of ankle sprains involve the lateral aspect of the ankle. The majority improve with non-surgical measures. Physiotherapy is useful and should be considered for a severe ankle sprain. If symptoms do not settle after 3 months, magnetic resonance imaging (MRI) scan/referral to secondary care is advised.

## Lesser toe deformities

## What are the common deformities of the lesser toes?

The most common deformities affecting the lesser toes are hammer toes, mallet toes and claw toes.

## What is a mallet toe?

Mallet toe is due to a flexion deformity of the distal interphalangeal (DIP) joint. It usually involves the longest lesser toe. It could be due to a congenital or developmental anomaly. The most common cause of an adult onset mallet toe is the lack of sufficient space for the longest toe in the shoe (Figure 8.21).

## What is a hammer toe?

Hammer toe is due to flexion deformity of the proximal interphalangeal (PIP) joint. Pressure caused by shoes leads to a callosity at the PIP joint. It can affect one or more toes. It is most commonly caused by mechanical factors such as flexion of the toe from an ill-fitting shoe or crowding from a significant hallux valgus deformity (Figure 8.22).

## What is a claw toe?

Claw toe deformity is defined as a toe where the primary deformity is a hyperextension deformity at the MTP joint. There is often a PIP joint flexion deformity as in hammer toes, but this is thought to be a secondary deformity. Claw toe deformity

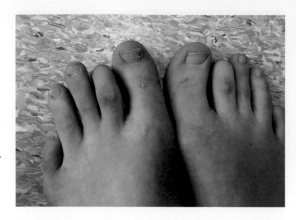

Figure 8.21 Bilateral second mallet toe deformity.

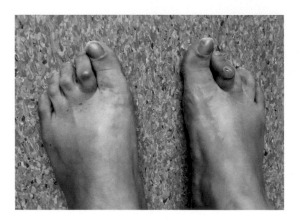

Figure 8.22 Bilateral hammer toe deformities affecting multiple toes.

usually can be associated with a neurological cause (e.g. Charcot–Marie–Tooth, peripheral neuropathy, compartment syndrome, diabetic neuropathy) or inflammatory cause (e.g. rheumatoid arthritis). In long-standing cases, the MTP joint dislocates (usually the second toe) resulting in callosity on the plantar aspect of the second metatarsal head (Figure 8.23a through c).

## What is bunionette deformity?

A bunionette deformity is also historically known as a *tailor's bunion* because of the tailor's crossed leg sitting position, which made the lateral aspect of the foot particularly prone to developing this problem.

A bunionette deformity is the rough equivalent of a hallux valgus deformity of the fifth toe.

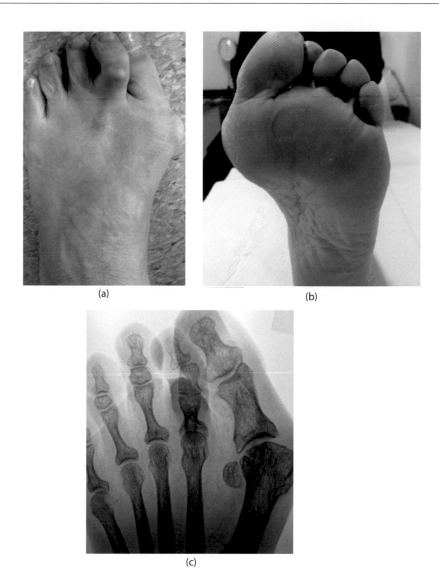

(a)

(b)

(c)

Figure 8.23 **(a)** Clawing with hammer toe deformity of second toe, **(b)** pressure callosity at second metatarsal head and **(c)** callosity due to the pressure caused by the second metatarsal head which is dislocated from the MTP joint as seen on x-rays.

The prominence of the lateral aspect of the fifth metatarsal head and/or a medial drift of the fifth toe proximal phalanx at the MTP joint results in a symptomatic protrusion on the lateral aspect of the foot.

## What is the treatment of a bunionette?

If wide-fitting shoes are not successful, surgical treatment can be considered. This involves a chevron osteotomy of the fifth metatarsal, which is fixed with a K wire. The K wire is removed at about 6 weeks. There is a good success rate of the surgical procedure to treat a bunionette.

## What is metatarsalgia?

Metatarsalgia indicates increased pressure on metatarsal heads (usually second or third). The most common cause is disparity in the length of metatarsals. This could be due to either a congenitally long second/third metatarsal or a shortened first metatarsal (following first ray surgery). The other

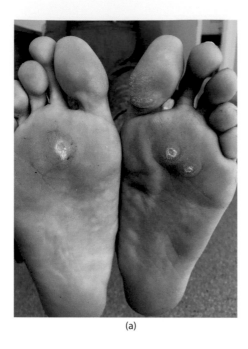
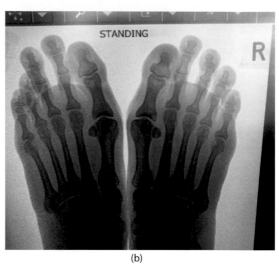

(a)

(b)

Figure 8.24 **(a)** Severe bilateral metatarsalgia and **(b)** x-rays showing short first metatarsal therefore resulting in increased pressure on second and third metatarsal heads leading to metatarsalgia.

important cause is synovitis of the MTP joint leading to subluxation or dislocation of the MTP joint. This could be due to an inflammatory pathology, trauma or secondary overload caused by a dysfunctional first ray. The soles should be inspected as in severe cases, there are visible callosities. Insoles (anterior arch support, metatarsal bar or metatarsal pad) are the first line of treatment. Surgical treatment in the form of metatarsal osteotomy could be considered in reluctant cases (Figure 8.24a and b).

## Less common but important foot and ankle problems

### What is Freiberg's disease?

This is due to reduced blood supply causing avascular necrosis of the metatarsal head. It usually involves the second metatarsal head. It is seen predominantly in women in the age group of 11–17 years. It presents as acute pain and swelling of the involved metatarsal head. It subsequently causes arthritis of the involved joint. The surgical treatment is in the form of debridement, removal of the loose body or osteotomy of the metatarsal. The prognosis of this condition is guarded (Figure 8.25).

### What is Sever's disease?

This is the most common cause of heel pain in children and adolescents. It is also called calcaneal apophysitis. It is a self-limiting, benign condition. It is due to repeated micro-trauma distal to insertion of the Achilles in a growing skeleton. The diagnosis is usually clinical. There is heel tenderness on palpation. It can be confused with plantar fasciitis. X-rays or an MRI scan can be considered to confirm the diagnosis. The treatment is reassurance, activity limitation and rest. If symptoms do not improve with these measures, then a plaster cast for 4–6 weeks can be considered. It does not require surgery.

### What is plantar fibroma?

This is the most common soft tissue lump in the sole. It is usually seen on the plantar aspect of the midfoot. It presents as swelling and can be associated with some discomfort secondary to pressure. Solitary plantar fibroma is a benign condition (Figure 8.26).

*Ledderhose's disease*, on the other hand, is referred to aggressive plantar fibromatosis

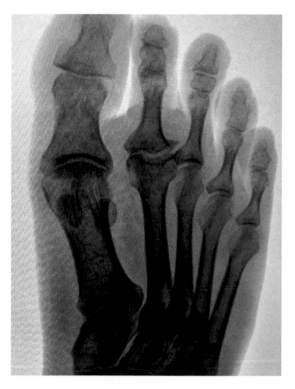

Figure 8.25 Freiberg's disease.

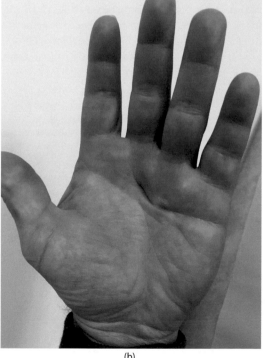

Figure 8.26 Plantar fibroma.

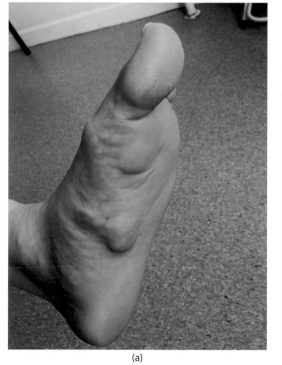

(a)

(b)

Figure 8.27 Ledderhose's disease: **(a)** aggressive plantar fibromatosis and **(b)** Dupuytren's contracture in same patient.

(Figure 8.27a) which could be associated with Dupuytren's contracture (Figure 8.27b) or *Peyronie disease*. This could be linked with genetic factors, chronic alcoholism, liver disease, epilepsy and diabetes.

Treatment in most cases is reassurance. In symptomatic cases, insoles or steroid injections are useful. Surgical treatment is usually not advised due to high risk of recurrence and wound healing problems.

## Painful swollen foot – what are the causes?

Once you have excluded infection (normal C-reactive protein [CRP]) and gout (normal uric acid), the most common cause of acute onset of pain and swelling of the foot is a stress fracture usually involving a metatarsal. The clinical examination will reveal swelling and marked bony tenderness. It can take 2–3 weeks for a stress fracture to show up on x-rays. Sometimes, x-rays do not show stress fractures, but there is persistent swelling and pain. In these cases, an MRI scan shows stress response or bone marrow oedema of a metatarsal or tarsal bone. Treatment is rest in a walking boot or plaster. In cases of recurrence, it is important to check Vitamin-D levels, conduct a DEXA scan to rule out osteoporosis or osteopenia and make sure that there is no significant foot deformity. A severe hindfoot varus can cause a stress fracture of the fifth metatarsal base, whereas a severe hallux valgus can lead to a stress fracture of the second or third metatarsals.

## What is Charcot foot?

This condition occurs in neuropathic (loss of or diminished sensation) feet. The most common cause is diabetes. Other causes include chronic alcoholism and peripheral neuropathy due to any other spinal/neurological problem. The midfoot is most commonly involved followed by the hindfoot, ankle and forefoot. The presentation is with marked redness, swelling and warmth. Pain might or might not be present. The key features of examination are raised local temperature and altered/diminished sensation. The peripheral pulses are usually palpable. There should be a high index of suspicion in patients with neuropathy. There are three stages of Charcot foot – acute, subacute and chronic. X-rays in initial stages might show no abnormality other than soft tissue swelling. Bone destruction is seen in later x-rays. If not diagnosed a and treated, this leads to significant deformity. These cases should be urgently referred to secondary care.

---

### SUMMARY POINTS

- Consider the possibility of Achilles rupture if a patient presents with a history of injury to the lower calf. The key words in the history are 'felt as if someone had kicked me'. The calf squeeze test is very sensitive and a good diagnostic tool. If in doubt, ask for an urgent ultrasound scan or specialist advice.
- Do not perform steroid injections for tendon problems in primary care.

## Acknowledgement

The author is grateful to Dr. Tom Rowley for reviewing this chapter and providing helpful comments from a primary care perspective.

## Resources

Bofas.org.uk
Aofas.org
footankleleicester.co.uk

## References

1. Soroceanu A, Sidhwa F, Aarabi S, Kaufman A, Glazebrook M. Surgical versus nonsurgical treatment of acute Achilles tendon rupture: A meta-analysis of randomized trials. *J Bone Joint Surg Am.* 2012;94(23):2136–2143.
2. Alfredson H. The chronic painful Achilles and patellar tendon: Research on basic biology and treatment. *Scand J Med Sci Sports.* 2005 Aug;15(4):252–259.
3. Bhatia M. Ankle arthritis: Review and current concepts. *J Arthroscopy Joint Surg.* 2014;1(1):19–26. http://dx.doi.org/10.1016/j.jajs.2013.11.001

4. Barg A, Zwicky L, Knupp M, Henninger HB, Hintermann B. Hintegra total ankle replacement: Survivorship analysis in 684 patients. *J Bone Joint Surg Am.* 2013 Jul 3;95(13): 1175–1183.

5. Baumhauer JF, Singh D, Glazebrook M, Blundell C, De Vries G, Le IL et al. Prospective, randomized, multi-centered clinical trial assessing safety and efficacy of a synthetic cartilage implant versus first metatarsophalangeal arthrodesis in advanced hallux rigidus. *Foot Ankle Int.* 2016 Feb 27;37(5):457–469. pii: 1071100716635560. [Epub ahead of print] PubMed PMID: 26922669.

6. Keene DJ, Alsousou J, Willett K. How effective are platelet rich plasma injections in treating musculoskeletal soft tissue injuries? *BMJ.* 2016;352:i517.

# 9

# Bone and soft tissue tumours/lumps and bumps

ROBERT U ASHFORD and PHILIP N GREEN

## Introduction

The general practitioner (GP) is often faced with patients with lumps and bumps. The causes of these are varied and can include herniae, cysts, benign and malignant soft tissue tumours and a plethora of other causes. This chapter covers musculoskeletal tumours as causes of lumps and bumps and aims to highlight when a GP should be worried. Benign soft tissue tumours are 100 times more common than soft tissue sarcomas (STSs), but it is important to recognise a potentially malignant soft tissue tumour. Delays in diagnosis result in tumour growth and the larger the primary tumour, the poorer the prognosis.[1]

## Soft tissue tumours

Red flag signs raise the possibility of potential malignancy. These have been thoroughly evaluated[2] and size is the most important.

The new National Institute for Health and Care Excellence (NICE) guidance NG12 (2015)[3] recommends urgent (within 2 weeks) ultrasound of all suspicious lumps and a very urgent (within 48 hours) time frame for those occurring in children and young people. The authors recommend the red flag signs (Table 9.1) continue to guide referral on a 2-week wait pathway, particularly if access to ultrasound is not available within that time period.

## Lipoma

### What is it?

A lipoma is a benign tumour of fat. Typically it is encapsulated and often subcutaneous, but it can

Table 9.1 Red and yellow flags for soft tissue sarcoma

| Red flag signs for soft tissue tumours |
|---|
| Larger than 4.3 cm (size of a golf ball) |
| Deep to deep fascia |
| Increasing in size |
| Painful |
| **Yellow flag sign (potentially concerning)** |
| Recurrence of a previously excised tumour |

occur either intramuscularly, submuscularly or even in bone.

### How does it present?

Lipomata usually present as a painless subcutaneous lump (Figure 9.1). When multiple, these can be painful (angiolipoma).

### What do I do?

If the lump is subcutaneous, an ultrasound is useful. Ultrasound is less helpful for deeper tumours, where magnetic resonance imaging (MRI) is the investigation of choice (Figure 9.2). Angiolipomata may have increased vascularity on ultrasound.

If there is atypia on ultrasound or other concerning features (see red flag signs), a 2-week wait (cancer pathway) referral for an STS should be made. Asymptomatic small superficial lipomata can be safely observed.

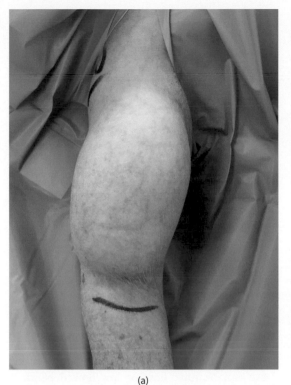
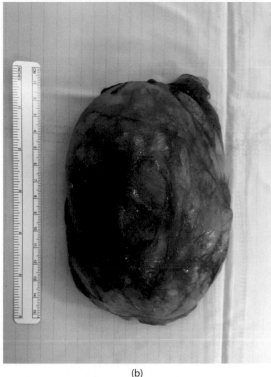

(a)

(b)

Figure 9.1 **(a)** Clinical photograph of large lipoma (larger than 4 cm) of the upper arm and (b) surgical specimen.

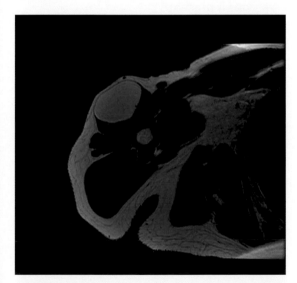

Figure 9.2 Magnetic resonance imaging (MRI) of subfascial lipoma.

### When should I be worried?

Concerning features are when lipomata exceed 4.3 cm (the size of a golf ball), when they are increasing in size, when there is a change in symptoms or if nodularity has developed. A 2-week wait referral should be made in these circumstances.

## Atypical lipomatous tumour

### What is it?

Atypical lipomatous tumours (ALTs) are a fatty tumour that are histologically different from straightforward benign lipomata. They usually occur in the periphery. The peak age incidence is 40–60 years. ALTs have the ability to dedifferentiate into liposarcomas and also have a higher incidence of recurrence than a normal lipoma. They only metastasise if they have undergone dedifferentiation. The term ALT is synonymous with well-differentiated liposarcoma (although well-differentiated liposarcoma is usually used to refer to those tumours in the retroperitoneum).

### How does it present?

ALTs present very much as for lipoma, usually a painless, often growing lump.

## What do I do?

The possibility of an ALT may be raised by imaging. Features on MRI include stranding or incomplete fat suppression. If the possibility has been raised on imaging then a referral to the sarcoma service is appropriate, rather than attempting to manage the patient in primary care.

If this diagnosis has been raised following minor surgery for excision of a lump, then the sarcoma service should once again be contacted for advice. In some cases, they may recommend surveillance or alternatively they may request the patient be formally referred for ongoing management.

ALTs do have the ability to dedifferentiate, and therefore, surgical excision will normally be the treatment of choice.

## When should I be worried?

The worrying features (red flag signs) of a benign lipoma apply equally to an ALT.

If a previously excised ALT recurs and is rapidly growing, then this may imply dedifferentiation and a 2-week wait sarcoma referral should be made.

## Ganglion/synovial cyst

### What is it?

A ganglion is a fluid-filled swelling arising from the lining of the tendon or a joint. They are most common around the wrist or the ankle.

### How does it present?

They usually present as a swelling overlying the joint that is fluctuant and can transilluminate. They can grow relatively large sometimes reaching in excess of 5 cm. They are usually painless unless compressing a nearby nerve.

### What do I do?

Normally, ganglia have typical appearances and the only reasons for concern are large size, rapid growth or the presence of unusual features.

The traditional remedy of hitting the ganglion with the family Bible is probably as effective as aspirating with a multineedle puncture; however, this technique risks damage to the surrounding structures.

If there are no symptoms other than unsightliness, ganglia can simply be observed.

When they occur at sites such as the proximal tibiofibular joint then nerve compression of the common peroneal nerve can occur and surgical treatment may be warranted. In this case, referral should be considered.

Immobilisation of a joint can cause resolution of swelling.

A radiograph may be necessary to confirm degenerative change and an ultrasound will usually clarify the lesion to be a ganglion.

### When should I be worried?

Recurrence after aspiration is an indication for referral. An MRI will sometimes be required prior to surgery (Figure 9.3).

## Haemangioma/arteriovenous malformation

### What is it?

A haemangioma or arteriovenous malformation is an abnormal collection of blood vessels. These can be high flow or low flow dependent on the feeding vasculature. An ultrasound can often be diagnostic.

### How does it present?

Subcutaneous and intramuscular haemangiomata can present as painful lumps. They may increase

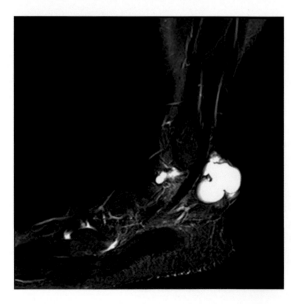

Figure 9.3 MRI scan of a multiloculated ganglion cyst of the ankle.

in size on exercise due to increased blood flow. Intramuscular haemangiomata can usually be compressed. Eighty percent of haemangiomata occur in patients under 30 years.

## What do I do?

Clinically, it may be difficult to determine their nature. An ultrasound, whilst very operator dependent, may be suggestive of a haemangioma, if the feeding vessel(s) can be determined.

Most haemangiomata are symptomatic, and therefore, referral to a soft tissue tumour service will be appropriate. An MRI will normally confirm the diagnosis and treatment options including sclerotherapy, embolization or surgical excision. These will usually be curative. Asymptomatic haemangiomata can be observed and may involute and undergo fatty replacement.

## When should I be worried?

The red flag signs of an STS again apply. It is virtually unheard of for haemangiomata to undergo malignant change. The challenge with them is diagnostics, and therefore, if features of concern for an STS are present then a 2-week wait referral to the sarcoma service should be made.

## Peripheral nerve sheath tumours: neurofibroma and schwannoma

### What is it?

A schwannoma is a benign neural tumour arising from a single fibre of a peripheral nerve, whereas a neurofibroma involves the nerve itself. Both can be multiple, neurofibromas often occurring within the disorder of neurofibromatosis and schwannomas as part of schwannomatosis.

### How does it present?

Both types of nerve tumour typically present with a small painful lump. On examination, there is likely to be a positive Tinel's sign (percussion of nerve elicits sensation of tinging in the distribution of the nerve) and pain on percussing. There can also be paraesthesia or weakness dependent on the size of the nerve and the peripheral nerve sheath tumour (PNST).

### What do I do?

Patients will normally be sufficiently symptomatic and excision will be merited. An MRI will usually confirm the diagnosis especially if the entering and exiting nerve is visualised (Figure 9.4).

Nerve tumours are often difficult to remove under a local anaesthetic because of their highly sensory nature, and therefore, excision under a general anaesthetic would normally be recommended.

### When should I be worried?

In the presence of neurofibromatosis, there is an incidence of PNSTs developing into malignant peripheral nerve sheath tumours (MPNSTs). Suspicion of this (typically rapid increase in size of

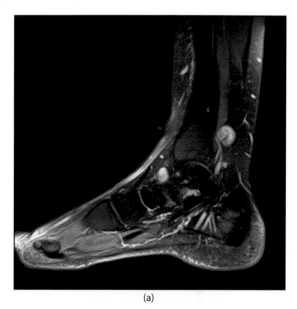

(a)

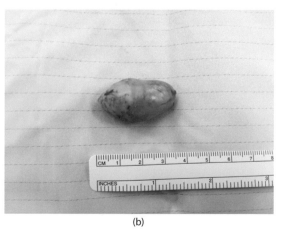

(b)

Figure 9.4 **(a)** MRI scan demonstrating two peripheral nerve sheath tumours (PNSTs) (schwannomata) and **(b)** clinical photograph of surgically resected PNST.

a neurofibroma) requires a referral into a sarcoma service. Deep neural lesions should also be referred.

## Soft tissue sarcomas

### What is it?

STSs are malignant tumours arising in the soft tissue. They represent approximately 1% of all malignant tumours. There are over 100 types in the most recent WHO classification. A detailed review of STSs is beyond the scope of this book.

### How does it present?

The typical presentation of an STS is of a painless mass that is increasing in size. Most are larger than 4.3 cm. They can occur at any age or in any part of the body. However, up to one-third of STSs can be small and superficial. (Figure 9.5).

### What do I do?

The most important thing is to recognise the possibility that a lesion is potentially an STS. In event of clinical suspicion, a 2-week wait referral should be made to the local sarcoma service or sarcoma diagnostic clinic. New NICE guidelines (2015) recommend an urgent ultrasound scan be obtained (<2 weeks for adults and 48 hours for children and young adults).

### When should I be worried?

Concerning features include when a lump is larger than 4.3 cm, deep to deep fascia, painful or increasing in size. The presence of all four of these red flag signs is associated with over an 80% chance that the lesion will be an STS.[2]

We strongly recommend that referral should not be delayed by investigation, as most of the investigations can be made expeditiously in the sarcoma centre (Figure 9.6).

For smaller superficial lesions where there is a lower degree of concern, an ultrasound scan is appropriate. In the event of an unexpected histological finding of an STS following excision in primary care, please refer to the section below on unexpected histology.

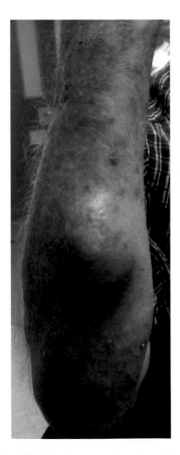

Figure 9.5 Clinical photograph of a soft tissue sarcoma (STS) of the forearm. The mass is firmer and fixed when compared to a lipoma.

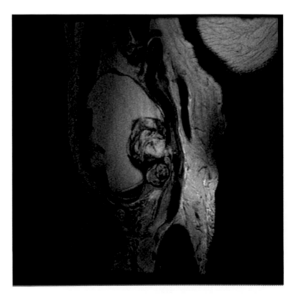

Figure 9.6 MRI of STS demonstrating all four red flag signs. The mass is deep, large, painful and growing. There is significant heterogeneity of the large mass on the MRI scan.

## The unexpected finding at minor surgery

Sometimes when undertaking minor surgery for a lump, the unexpected will be encountered. This commonly occurs when a presumed lipoma or cyst is being removed and on incising the skin, the consistency of the tumour is obviously not that of a lipoma. In these circumstances, the following measures should be taken:

1. Do not panic.
2. Take a generous biopsy of the lesion but do not remove it all (in the event it turns out to be a sarcoma, it is easier to re-resect if the tumour can be palpated).
3. Secure haemostasis and close the wound.
4. Mark the histology 'URGENT? SARCOMA' – this should ensure the pathology goes to the correct histopathologist.
5. It is useful at this stage to contact the clinical nurse specialist at the local sarcoma centre to flag the patient to the sarcoma service.
6. A plan should be made to review the patient early to enable expeditious referral.

If the histology does confirm a sarcoma, then an appropriate 2-week wait referral should be made. The sarcoma team is likely to be aware of the patient via the pathologist. The patient must be informed of the diagnosis (it is unhelpful if the first realization the patients have that they have cancer is when they arrive in an oncology clinic). They should be made aware they are likely to need both further (staging) investigations and further surgery. This enables sensible discussions regarding management to happen in the sarcoma clinic.

### Unexpected histology of a soft tissue sarcoma

If the lump has been excised during minor surgery, and the histology comes back unexpectedly as a sarcoma, then the sarcoma team will often already be aware of the diagnosis through the reporting pathologist referring the patient to a multidisciplinary team (MDT). A 2-week referral wait should also be made to a sarcoma clinic. The patient should be informed of the diagnosis. Accompanying the 2-week referral, a copy of both the operation note and the histopathology report should be enclosed. It is further advisable to telephone the CNS at the regional sarcoma centre (details can be found via the British Sarcoma Group website, www.british-sarcomagroup.org.uk) to facilitate referral and early review.

The patients should be warned that they should expect to undergo additional investigations and then further surgery. This enables the sarcoma team to directly request further imaging (communication with the CNS as above can facilitate this).

It is imperative to inform the patients of the diagnosis so that they are able to make sensible management decisions at the time of their consultation. Furthermore, a full blood count (FBC) and urea and electrolytes (U&E) tests should be performed if there are no recent results (this prevents delays and will enable contrast enhanced imaging to be undertaken).

## The rarer soft tissue tumour

## Pigmented villonodular synovitis/diffuse-type tenosynovial giant cell tumour

### What is it?

Pigmented villonodular synovitis (PVNS) is a benign progressive lesion that arises from the lining of a synovium causing it to thicken and overgrow.

### How does it present?

It typically occurs in one of two forms – nodular (localised) or diffuse. It can cause joint pain, swelling and stiffness. The nodular form can result in locking and symptoms can be very acute. Untreated, PVNS can cause joint destruction and arthritis.

### What do I do?

Plain radiograph and/or ultrasound may raise the possibility of an intra-articular lesion and an MRI scan may further highlight the possibility of PVNS. A tissue diagnosis is, however, necessary for confirmation.

PVNS should be managed by the sarcoma service and will typically be investigated by a biopsy prior to surgical excision.

There are major differences between the two types of PVNS in terms of treatment and local recurrence, with the nodular form being easier to excise and having a lower recurrence rate.

### When should I be worried?

PVNS does not undergo malignant degeneration, but symptoms may mimic a sarcoma.

In the event of concern, a 2-week wait referral to the sarcoma service is mandatory, otherwise simply referring to one of the sarcoma orthopaedic surgeons on suspicion or confirmation of diagnosis is recommended.

## Desmoid fibromatosis/aggressive fibromatosis

### What is it?

This is a very rare tumour-like condition, the management of which can be extremely challenging.

### How does it present?

Desmoid fibromatosis can present very much as an STS with a large progressive mass most commonly in the limb girdle.

### What do I do?

As with all progressive large masses, a 2-week wait sarcoma referral should be made. Whilst the referral is happening, a similar request can be submitted for an ultrasound, but again this is very operator dependent.

MRI and biopsy will be required to confirm the diagnosis.

In females using oestrogen contraceptive pills, where there is a confirmed diagnosis of desmoid fibromatosis, it would normally be recommended that these be changed to progesterone-only pills.

### When should I be worried?

Desmoid fibromatosis is normally a diagnosis made following referral of a suspected STS, and therefore, a 2-week wait STS referral should be made.

## Bone tumours

## Osteochondroma (exostosis)

### What is it?

These are benign bony swellings that have continuity with the medullary cavity and a cartilaginous cap. They can be either sessile or pedunculated. They usually become obvious in childhood and arise from the surface of bone, near the growth plate.

### How does it present?

Osteochondromata present as a bony lump which may or may not be increasing in size. The lump is usually painless and close to a joint. Large osteochondromata may be associated with pain on exercise with a snapping of the fibrous tissues over the top of the osteochondroma. Unusually sited osteochondromata (e.g. popliteal fossa, Figure 9.7) can be associated with paraesthesia or alteration in blood flow. These are rarer.

### What do I do?

A plain radiograph will normally be diagnostic (Figure 9.7).

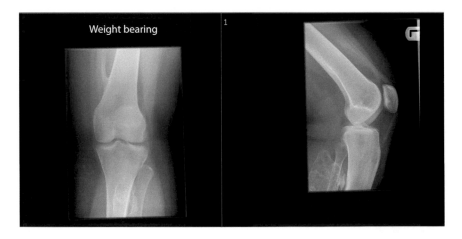

Figure 9.7 Radiograph of large popliteal fossa exostosis arising from fibula with further pedunculated exostosis from medial distal femur. The patient has hereditary multiple exostoses.

Osteochondromata are either sessile (broad based) or pedunculated (narrow stalk).

## When should I be worried?

If an osteochondroma becomes symptomatic after the patient has reached skeletal maturity, either in terms of an increase in size or symptoms (pain), then these are concerning features. Orthopaedic referral is indicated for either of these symptoms.

Features of concern for potential malignant transformation of an osteochondroma are growth after skeletal maturity or pain without trauma in a previously painless bony lump.

In the event that a known exostosis/osteochondroma is increasing in size, an up-to-date plain radiograph is necessary and an ultrasound or MRI scan is useful to assess the thickness of the cartilaginous cap. Thickness in excess of 1.5 cm would be worrying for chondrosarcomatous change.

Surgical excision is usually indicated for symptomatic osteochondromata.

# Enchondroma

## What is it?

An enchondroma is a benign cartilaginous tumour occurring within the bone.

## How does it present?

Enchondromata are usually painless. When they occur in the hands or feet, they can cause deformity. They can be multiple (*Ollier disease or Maffucci syndrome*) and can sometimes cause pain.

## What do I do?

Plain radiographs will usually be diagnostic. If imaging is diagnostic of an enchondroma and the patient is asymptomatic, then treatment may not be necessary and simply observation will suffice. If there are features of concern, then an orthopaedic referral is indicated.

Asymptomatic lesions should be observed with interval plain radiographs (approximately 1-year intervals to ensure stability over 2 years, and thereafter, if it becomes symptomatic).

## When should I be worried?

Pain associated with an enchondroma is worrying for sarcomatous dedifferentiation. Radiological features of concern include alteration in the bone cortex, destruction of the bone, a soft tissue mass and an enchondroma occupying the width of the medullary cavity. These features are worrying for chondrosarcomatous change and a 2-week wait referral should be made.

# Multiple bone lesions

## What is it?

Multiple bone lesions usually fall into one of five categories. They are multiple osteochondromas (multiple hereditary exostoses [MHEs]/diaphyseal aclasis) (Figure 9.7), multiple enchondromata (Ollier disease or Maffucci syndrome), fibrous dysplasia, Paget's disease and skeletal metastases.[4]

Exostoses and enchondromata have been discussed earlier. There is potential for malignant change in both multiple osteochondroma and enchondroma, with differentiation in Ollier and Maffucci being more common and some reports suggesting in Maffucci it is as high as 100%.

Fibrous dysplasia can be polyostotic or monostotic. It commonly affects the long bones of young adults. The classic radiological appearance of a pagetic femur is of a shepherd's crook deformity. There is a broadened diaphysis and a ground glass appearance.

Monostotic fibrous dysplasia is a more indolent condition. Polyostotic fibrous dysplasia associated with precocious puberty and café au lait spots is synonymous with McCune–Albright syndrome. This has increased risk of malignant transformation compared with the monostotic subtype.

For MHE and multiple enchondromata, a pelvic radiograph should be obtained at diagnosis. This is because pelvic lesions with sarcomatous change can present late if one is unaware of them. Known pelvic lesions can be observed to allow early detection of malignant degeneration.

# Osteoid osteoma/osteoblastoma

## What is it?

Osteoid osteoma and osteoblastomas are small, bone-forming benign lesions which are normally present in either a juxta-cortical or intramedullary location.

## How does it present?

The textbook presentation for an osteoid osteoma is night pain which is alleviated by non-steroidal anti-inflammatory drugs (NSAIDs). The difference between the two is simply size, with osteoblastomas being larger than 2 cm. The tibia is the most common location for an osteoid osteoma. Twenty-five percent of osteoblastomas occur in the spine.

## What do I do?

A plain radiograph will often raise the possibility of a sclerotic lesion surrounded by a small nidus.

In the event that a plain radiograph is suggestive of an osteoid osteoma, then a trial on non-steroidals is a usual diagnostic entity. Referral to a local bone tumour unit is appropriate, where the diagnosis is often confirmed with a fine-cut computed tomography (CT) and a biopsy. Treatment is by simple analgesia in the first instance. Recalcitrant tumours can be treated by radiofrequency or laser ablation, unless the location precludes it. In these cases, surgical curettage or excision is appropriate.

## When should I be worried?

These are benign tumours and do not undergo malignant change. If there are radiological features of concern, a sarcoma 2-week wait referral should be made.

## Fibrous cortical defect/non-ossifying fibroma

### What is it?

This is a benign fibrous cortical lesion which often appears as a lytic lesion on plain radiograph.

### How does it present?

Almost invariably, these are an incidental finding when a trivial injury occurs. The history is usually of a sprain during sport in a child or young adult. Attendance of the emergency department precipitates imaging of the injured area, and the lesion is usually identified on the plain radiographs. Fibrous cortical defect (FCD) and non-ossifying fibroma (NOF) are interchangeable terms. They sometimes occur in multiple sites and are most common in adolescents.

### What do I do?

In the event that a radiograph has been organised in primary care and shows an FCD, it will normally require no more than surveillance imaging. These lesions usually spontaneously resolve.

FCD can predispose to pathological fracture, but this is rare. Large lesions require ongoing surveillance to exclude progression.

### When should I be worried?

Pain associated with an FCD is unusual.

If pain is over the ankle ligament for example, then it is unlikely to be related to the FCD, but if the pain is bony, then an orthopaedic referral is mandatory.

Patients with known FCD, who develop increased symptoms, require up-to-date imaging and orthopaedic review.

## Bone cysts – unicameral (simple) bone cyst/aneurysmal bone cyst

### What is it?

These are benign bone tumours that predominantly occur in children. A unicameral bone cyst (UBC) (synonymous with simple bone cyst) is a fluid-filled cavity within the bone that primarily occurs in childhood and adolescence. UBCs usually affect long bones.

An aneurysmal bone cyst (ABC) is a solitary blood-filled fibrous lined cavity that expands the bone.

### How does it present?

Most UBCs are discovered after a pathological fracture or when a radiograph is performed for an unrelated problem. UBCs are one of the most common benign bone tumours in children and occur more frequently in boys than girls.

ABCs often present with pain and swelling during the teenage years but can occur at any age, and account for between 1% and 6% of benign bone tumours. ABCs should be referred to a paediatric orthopaedic or bone tumour service. About 80% of ABCs occur in patients under 20 years of age. They can occur secondarily to other bone tumours particularly giant cell tumours (GCTs).

### What do I do?

If the patient presents with a pathological fracture, they will normally be managed by the trauma service, usually with observation whilst the fracture heals.

If a bone cyst presents as an incidental finding, then an orthopaedic referral to a paediatric orthopaedic surgeon is indicated.

Once a child is fully grown, it is normal for UBCs to heal.

ABCs usually require surgical intervention, often in the form of curettage.

### When should I be worried?

If the imaging is not clear cut and a UBC is only a differential diagnosis, then referral should be made to establish an accurate diagnosis. All ABCs on imaging should be referred.

## Giant cell tumour of bone

### What is it?

GCT of bone is a rare locally aggressive but benign bone tumour that occurs in the epiphysis of the long bones, usually between the ages of 20 and 40 years. GCTs are rare in children or over those aged 65 years.

### How does it present?

Usually these will present with pain over the bone, and pain on movement of the joint that increases with activity. There may be a mass present, and the pain is usually progressive. They may, however, present as a pathological fracture.

### What do I do?

Typically, giant cell tumours present with pain that is progressive and unremitting. A plain radiograph would normally be diagnostic showing a lytic juxta-articular lesion.

The presence of a giant cell tumour in the bone requires an urgent 2-week wait referral to the local bone sarcoma service. It is helpful to check the calcium and serum parathyroid hormone level because a brown tumour of hyperparathyroidism has identical radiological features.

An MRI scan and a biopsy would normally be necessary to confirm the diagnosis.

### When should I be worried?

If extensive destruction is reported on the plain radiograph, then there is imminent risk of pathological fracture. Some bone sarcomas can mimic giant cell tumours, and a biopsy will be required for diagnosis. All imaging diagnosed giant cell tumours should be referred as a 2-week wait to a bone tumour centre.

## Primary bone sarcomas

### What is it?

Bone sarcomas are a very rare form of cancer arising in bone. They include osteosarcoma, chondrosarcoma, Ewing's sarcoma and spindle cell sarcoma of bone. There are approximately 550 new primary bone sarcomas in the United Kingdom per annum.

### How does it present?

Primary bone sarcomas often present in teenagers and young adults with unexplained progressive bone pain or a palpable mass. The pain may have been present for many months. The pain may be unaffected by activity. Any mass may be painful or painless.

### What do I do?

A plain radiograph is normally diagnostic. This should be arranged expeditiously in the event that a primary bone sarcoma is considered as a differential diagnosis. The suspicion of a primary bone sarcoma on radiology will normally be flagged to the local orthopaedic team or orthopaedic oncology service. In the event that this has not happened, a 2-week wait sarcoma referral is mandatory.

Delays in diagnosis can be detrimental to the patient's outcome.

### When should I be worried?

Unremitting progressive pain particularly at night or unrelated to activity should raise the suspicion of a bone sarcoma. Similarly, a bony mass should raise suspicion and in these circumstances, urgent radiographs should be arranged. The referrer should chase the results of these so that delays in referral are avoided.

At the time of referral, the patient (and parents if appropriate) should be made aware of the possible diagnosis and have the expectation that a number of further investigations will be necessary. If sarcoma is confirmed, the patient will be referred to National Bone Tumour Centres for treatment, which in England are situated at Stanmore, Birmingham, Oxford, Oswestry and Newcastle.

## Skeletal metastases

### What is it?

These are malignant tumours that are the result of a primary cancer spreading to the bone. They can be sclerotic (bone forming) or lytic (bone resorbing) or mixed. The most common cancers to spread to bone are breast, lung, thyroid, kidney and prostate.

### How does it present?

Skeletal metastases can present as either bone pain, pathological fracture or with signs of nerve root compression. Hypercalcaemia can also be a manifestation of metastatic bone disease.

### What do I do?

The presence of new bone pain or new spinal symptoms in a patient with bone malignancy should raise the possibility of a diagnosis of skeletal metastases.

In the event that there is primary care access to a staging CT, then this is often the first line of investigation, although a plain radiograph may be diagnostic.

For a primary tumour such as prostate cancer, measuring the tumour markers may provide evidence of relapse.

When the suspicion of a skeletal metastasis has been raised, the serum calcium should be checked (as well as other routine bloods including an FBC).

The patient should be referred back to the primary tumour MDT and to the primary managing oncologist as a matter of urgency.

If the suspicion of skeletal metastases has been raised without a known primary, then a referral to a cancer of unknown primary (CUP) team, or a discussion with a local orthopaedic surgeon regarding appropriateness of referral, should be made.

### When should I be worried?

New neurological signs may suggest, in a patient with previous cancer, imminent metastatic spinal cord compression (MSCC) and urgent referral to the MSCC service should be undertaken. This is normally through an MSCC coordinator who can facilitate all the above investigations.

## SUMMARY

The ratio of benign to malignant soft tissue lumps is 100:1, and the majority of lumps that are seen in general practice will turn out to be benign lipomas, ganglia and the like.

However, suspicious features such as red flag signs (Table 9.1) should mandate a 2-week wait sarcoma referral. Recent NICE guidelines recommend urgent ultrasound assessment on all worrying lumps.

If there is a suspicion of bone malignancy, then a plain radiograph is mandatory prior to referral as this will often be diagnostic. Growing pains are a diagnosis of exclusion and the presence of persistent bone pain in a child should raise the possibility of a bone sarcoma.

Clinicians within sarcoma services are amenable to providing advice and with the advent of picture archiving and communication system (PACS) and image sharing, images can be reviewed with relative ease.

Regional bone and STS services will normally have contact details available via the GP intranet for individual regions. All bone and STS services can be identified from the British Sarcoma Group website at www.britishsarcomagroup.org.uk

Two-week wait sarcoma referrals should contain the following information:

- Patient demographic and contact details
- Symptoms and signs
- Comorbidities
- Radiology reports
- Operation notes (if appropriate)
- Histology reports (if appropriate)

For clearly worrying bone or soft tissue lesions, undertaking the following bloods facilitate the arrangement of further investigations: FBC, U&E and clotting.

# References

1. Grimer RJ. Size matters for sarcomas! *Ann R Coll Surg Engl.* 2006;88(6):519.
2. Nandra R, Forsberg J, Grimer R. If your lump is bigger than a golf ball and growing, think sarcoma. *Eur J Surg Oncol.* 2015;41(10):1400–1405.
3. NICE. Suspected cancer: Recognition and referral. (NG12). 2015, https://www.nice.org.uk/guidance/ng12
4. Muthusamy S, Conway S, Temple HT. Five polyostotic conditions that general orthopaedic surgeons should recognize (or should not miss). *Orthop Clin North Am.* 2014;45(3):417–429.

# 10

# Preoperative fitness and perioperative issues in MSK patients

RALPH LEIGHTON and STEPHEN LE MAISTRE

## Introduction

There is no doubt that surgery is increasingly being offered to patients who only a few years ago would have been declined surgery on 'medical' or 'anaesthetic' grounds. Whilst the identification and improved management of such higher risk patients has enabled this change, it has also become an almost self-fulfilling prophecy leading to the boundaries of practice shifting further and further. The challenge now is to successfully manage our whole patient population appropriately within the constraints of available resources.

## Preoperative assessment

Preoperative assessment is an imperfect science; screening is now generally undertaken in nurse-led clinics though more and more trusts now have consultant-led clinics for the higher risk patients to attend.

Many patients will now attend a pre-assessment clinic in advance of their surgery. This visit serves several purposes (assessment of fitness, ordering and obtaining investigations and providing preoperative instructions and in some cases medication). Patients should be reminded of the importance of attending.

There are essentially two key questions when assessing 'fitness' for surgery:

1. Does the patient have sufficient physiological capacity to cope with the surgical insult and the perioperative stress response?
2. Have any comorbidities been optimised in order to maximise this capacity?

We would also add that these questions should ideally be addressed before discussing with the patient the relative risks of surgery to them.

## Assessment of physiological capacity

Exercise capacity can be usefully assessed by the use of metabolic equivalent tasks (METs).

| Task | METs |
| --- | --- |
| Watching TV | 1 |
| Walking slowly | 3 |
| Climbing stairs | 4 |
| Cycling slowly | 4 |
| Jogging | 7 |

Generally speaking, four METs equate to climbing a flight of stairs without difficulty, walking steadily without limitation. If patients can manage four METs activity, then this is very reassuring, and it is unlikely that they will benefit from extensive preoperative cardiorespiratory investigation.

However, exercise tolerance is very difficult to measure objectively in the orthopaedic surgical population and thus it comes down to careful history taking and clinical experience.

If arthritis or other comorbidity precludes active exertion, then formal investigation of cardiopulmonary exercise tolerance may be indicated. This is only rarely carried out for minor (e.g. carpal tunnel) or intermediate (e.g. primary joint repair) surgery.

Cardiopulmonary exercise testing (CPET) is considered by many to be the gold standard investigation of perioperative fitness and is available in many (but not most) hospitals in the United Kingdom. Patients undertake a short period of supervised and defined exercise either on a treadmill, exercise bike or hand crank machine. This test gives an excellent estimation of the patient's physiological capacity and their ability to weather the perioperative period (Figure 10.1).

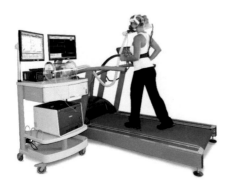

Figure 10.1 Cardiopulmonary exercise testing.

## Optimising patients with significant comorbidity

There are many diseases and disease processes that could or may affect surgery and anaesthesia. The basic principle is that these should be as optimally managed as possible before undertaking elective surgery.

## Specific systems

1. The diabetic patient
2. Cardiovascular disease
3. Respiratory disease and sleep apnoea
4. Obesity
5. Anaesthesia-specific issues

## The diabetic patient

Guidelines[1] relating to the perioperative management of the diabetic patient would suggest that:

- Diabetes affects up to 10% of all surgical patients.
- Diabetic patients suffer from increased mortality, morbidity and length of stay.
- All referrals for surgery contain a minimum data set (Appendix 12 of the guidance).
- If patients have chronically poor control, they should be referred to the diabetic team.

The impact of this is that patients with suboptimal control may be cancelled at pre-assessment or on the day of surgery and they should be warned of this.

## Cardiovascular disease and ischaemic heart disease

There are established guidelines for investigation of ischemic heart disease in the surgical patient.[2] Broadly speaking, patients with good physiological capacity and stable symptoms do not merit any specific investigation.

Patients with recent myocardial infarction or recent cardiac stenting are at dramatically increased risks of cardiac events during elective surgery. These risks reduce (but are still elevated) after 6 months.

## Valve disease

Valve disease is not uncommon in those aged 65 years and over. It is still likely that in most units that if a new murmur is detected at pre-assessment, the surgery will be deferred until this has been investigated. Therefore, it is worthwhile exercise to exclude the presence of a cardiac murmur at the point of referral for surgery. Echocardiograms instigated in the community are often not available to the hospital.

## Hypertension

Pre-existing significant hypertension leads to cardiovascular instability during anaesthesia and increases morbidity and mortality. It is not clear that moderate pre-existing hypertension is directly linked to increased morbidity or mortality. It is not surprising therefore that this is a somewhat controversial area of preoperative management. In general, patients with a systolic >180 mmHg or diastolic >110 mmHg should have their surgery postponed to allow for adequate control of their hypertension.[3]

## Respiratory disease

Respiratory disease is best managed by assessment of the patient's functional status. Investigations such as chest x-ray and spirometry are not predictive of respiratory complications postoperatively. As with other systems, the essential question is whether the patient's respiratory function can be further optimised before surgery.

## Sleep apnoea

Sleep apnoea is not uncommon in the surgical population and does not in itself preclude surgery. Additional precautions are required and the anaesthetist may well ask for a formal assessment by a sleep clinic prior to elective surgery.

## Obesity

Obesity is increasingly common in the surgical population. Whilst weight loss might reduce the need and risks of surgery, it is often unrealistic to expect significant weight loss prior to surgery particularly if the operation is for painful arthritis. The patients should be warned that their obesity will be referred to by hospital medical staff and that they may have an altered treatment pathway as a result. It is helpful to include the patient's body mass index (BMI) on any referral for surgery as it may trigger enhanced preoperative screening.

## Anaesthesia-specific issues

Whilst none of these issues are normally diagnosed in the community, it is important that they are flagged during any referral for surgery.

## The difficult airway

The patient may have had a prior anaesthetic and been issued with an 'airway alert'. If this is the case, a copy should be sent with any referral for surgery.

## Malignant hyperthermia

This is a rare inherited condition which presents significant challenges at the time of surgery. All first-degree relatives should be tested.

## Suxamethonium (or 'scoline') apnoea

This is an inherited deficiency in plasma cholinesterase which leads to prolonged duration of action of some muscle relaxants. This is of no significant consequence if appropriately identified. It is often incorrectly labelled as an 'allergy to'. All first-degree relatives should be tested.

## Allergy

Allergy to anaesthetics agents is well described. Often the trigger agent is difficult to identify because of the rapid coadministration of drugs during anaesthesia. In virtually all cases alternative agents can be used for future anaesthetics.

## The anaesthetic itself

The actual method of anaesthesia varies widely between operations and between hospitals. Broadly speaking, operations can be carried out as follows:

- With general anaesthesia ± local or regional anaesthesia
- With regional anaesthesia ± sedation
- With local anaesthesia ± sedation

Unfortunately, patients rarely get to meet the anaesthetist prior to the day of surgery and thus can be very nervous about any or all of the above options.

The Royal College of Anaesthetists has a wide range of patient information leaflets which are available at http://www.rcoa.ac.uk/patientinfo.

Broadly speaking, the overall risks of regional (spinal/epidural) and general anaesthesia are similar in the 'whole population' and different anaesthetists have differing preferences for how to manage certain operations. For high-risk patients, it is more likely that a regional anaesthetic is recommended.

## Postoperative issues (presenting to the GP)

As described above, surgery and anaesthesia are associated with massive physiological challenges and changes followed by an acute stress reaction. It is therefore not surprising that this leads to occasional problems in some patients.

With patients being discharged earlier following surgery, these are more likely to present in the community. In general terms, all hospitals will have a consultant anaesthetist on call who can be contacted if you have a concern about a postoperative anaesthesia complication.

1. *Acute coronary syndrome:* Cardiac events and troponin rises following surgery are well described and should be proactively managed as in the non-surgical population. Recent surgery does not preclude cardiological management, and these patients should be dealt with by urgent referral to hospital or cardiology as per your usual management of the non-surgical patient.
2. *Cognitive dysfunction*: Cognitive dysfunction[4] following surgery in common in the elderly population (1:4 at 1 week, 1:10 at 6 months). There is no specific investigation or treatment other than to exclude other causes of cognitive impairment which have been unmasked by anaesthesia.
3. *Headache (following regional anaesthesia)*: Post-dural puncture headache occurs not uncommonly in 0.5%–2% patients who have had a regional anaesthetic. Meningitis is reported following spinal/epidural anaesthesia but is very rare.

Should a patient present following surgery with a headache and features such as photophobia, neck stiffness, postural component, tinnitus or neurological signs or are unwell, they should be urgently referred back to the treating hospital as serious side effects can occur.

4. *Neurological symptoms*: Nerve damage following regional anaesthesia is rare (1:1000 or less) and usually resolves. The incidence of permanent nerve injury is estimated at 1:40,000. If patients present with neurological symptoms, they should be discussed with the relevant anaesthetic department. Any patient presenting with vertebral canal symptoms needs immediate referral to a spinal centre.
5. *Sore throat*: A postoperative sore throat occurs in 20%–40% of patients who have had a general anaesthetic and usually resolves within 72 hours.
6. *Awareness*: Awareness occurs in around 1:19,000 anaesthetics (though less commonly in orthopaedic surgery). Any patient report of awareness should be discussed with the relevant anaesthetic department so that they can arrange appropriate follow-up.

## SUMMARY POINTS

1. Comorbidities should be optimised before surgery.
2. Physiological capacity is the most important predictor of perioperative complications.
3. Diabetic patients suffer from increased mortality, morbidity and length of stay.
4. Post-anaesthesia complications should be discussed with the relevant anaesthetic department.

### Resources

Introduction to CPEX, https://www.youtube.com/watch?v=U_0Gi0gozgU

### Image source and licence

https://commons.wikimedia.org/wiki/File: Ergospirometry_laboratory.jpg?uselang=en-gb

# References

1. Ketan D, Daniel F, Louise H, Anne K, Nicholas L, Gerry R et al. Management of adults with diabetes undergoing surgery and elective procedures: Improving standards. April 2011, http://www.diabetologists-abcd.org.uk/JBDS/JBDS_IP_Surgery_Adults_Full.pdf

2. Fleisher LA, Fleischmann KE, Auerbach AD, Barnason SA, Beckman JA, Bozkurt B et al. 2014 ACC/AHA guideline on perioperative cardiovascular evaluation and management of patients undergoing noncardiac surgery. *J Am Coll Cardiol*. 2014;64(22):e77–e137. doi:10.1016/j.jacc.2014.07.944

3. Keith A, Iain W. *Oxford Handbook of Anaesthesia*. Oxford: Oxford University Press, 2011.

4. Deiner S, Silverstein JH. Postoperative delirium and cognitive dysfunction. *Br J Anaesth*. 2009;103 (Suppl 1):i41–i46.

# 11

# Rheumatology for general practitioners

KEHINDE SUNMBOYE and ASH SAMANTA

## Introduction

Rheumatology covers a wide range of clinical conditions. There are some that directly overlap with orthopaedics, for example soft-tissue tendinitis or ligamentous conditions, osteoarthritis (OA) or 'chronic' low back pain. The underlying pathogenesis of these is usually 'mechanical' in nature. There are other conditions that fall principally within the domain of rheumatology, typically such as rheumatoid arthritis (RA) or systemic lupus erythematosus (SLE). The pathogenesis of these usually involves an immunological basis along with a systemic inflammatory process.

Patients, however, do not present to the primary care clinician with clearly attached diagnostic labels. They present with symptoms which are mainly articular and which overlap with conditions that could be orthopaedic or rheumatological in nature. The challenge therefore is to accurately diagnose or recognise what is or might be affecting the patient, so that an optimal referral and care pathway may be effected.

In this chapter, we have limited ourselves to those commonly occurring conditions that are best managed through a rheumatology service. We have attempted to provide key practical pointers through the lens of a clinician in a busy general practice setting that might assist a general practitioner (GP) in best managing the patient who presents with musculoskeletal symptoms. In doing so, the authors have drawn upon their own clinical expertise over several years, and have presented this in a format of key issues that need to be considered to facilitate diagnosis and a management plan that is principally rheumatology based.

The reader might also wish to consult Sukaini et al. (2014) which provides a general overview.

## Rheumatoid arthritis

## What is important in the history?

It is important to ascertain the duration of joint symptoms, which joints are affected and whether there has been any joint swelling associated with pain.

The joints involved in RA are typically the small joints. There is symmetrical involvement of hands, wrist and feet. Bilateral large joint involvement can also be in conjunction with the aforementioned joints. Joint pain and swelling is usually present early in the disease course. Early morning stiffness, if greater than 1 hour, is considered significant of an inflammatory process.

Continuous presence of symptoms for greater than 6 weeks is significant and reflects that it isn't a transient process. Family history of RA increases the likelihood of RA in the patient, based on various gene studies.

It is also pertinent to check for a history of psoriasis and inflammatory bowel disease which are important causes of inflammatory arthritis to rule out and exclude.

## What focused examination will help to make the diagnosis?

A general examination is undertaken initially to assess the patient's overall condition.

Puffiness or swelling between the metacarpal heads with loss of the gaps between the metacarpal heads is a sign of early synovial inflammation. Metacarpophalangeal (MCP) and metatarsophalangeal (MTP) 'squeeze' tests are important, even if synovitis is not clinically evident. A positive pain response may suggest underlying synovial inflammation when gentle pressure is applied and the patient feels pain.

Any of the affected joints with symptoms should be assessed if synovitis is clinically evident (site of swelling, range of movement, tenderness, periarticular structures and deformities).

## What key investigations should I do?

The full blood count (FBC) may show *normocytic normochromic anaemia* related to persistent inflammation ('anaemia of chronic disease'). *Thrombocytosis* may also be seen which usually suggests ongoing inflammation.

Inflammatory markers such as *C-reactive protein* (CRP), *plasma viscosity* (PV) or *erythrocyte sedimentation rate* (ESR) may be increased. Elevations of these markers usually reflect underlying inflammation. It should be remembered that inflammatory markers may not always be elevated, particularly in early disease or if there is very low-grade inflammation.

The presence of *rheumatoid factor* (RF) and *anti-citrullinated peptide antibodies* (anti-CCP) may help in providing a guide to the severity and prognosis of RA. RF is found in approximately 70% of patients with RA. Patients who are negative for RF are referred to as *seronegative*. A patient who is seronegative and who has an inflammatory arthropathy may have either seronegative RA, or one of the forms of seronegative spondyloarthropathy (as described later in this chapter). Anti-CCP antibodies when positive are highly suggestive of RA and have a specificity of over 90%.

X-rays of the affected joint may show erosions, if symptoms have been present for more than 6 months. Erosions may be seen early at the ulnar styloid. An ultrasound of the affected joints is useful to assess for synovitis especially when not clinically evident and is more helpful for superficial joints but request should not delay referral.

## How do I manage this condition?

Patients need urgent referral to a rheumatologist, because early treatment ensures better long-term outcomes. Non-steroidal anti-inflammatory drugs (NSAIDs) can be used initially whilst patients await specialist review. Oral or intramuscular steroids should be used only after specialist advice.

## What early clinical features will help in making the diagnosis?

- Bilateral symmetrical small joint arthropathy (hands or feet)
- Positive squeeze tests in MCP and MTP joints
- Presence of synovitis in any of the joints

## When should I refer for a specialist opinion?

Patients should be referred as soon as diagnosis is suspected based on clinical features.

## Common pitfalls and how can I avoid these?

Lack of clinically evident synovitis does not sufficiently exclude RA as the likely diagnosis. These patient groups will often need ultrasound scanning to rule out RA. Negative CRP, PV and ESR do not always exclude RA as the diagnosis. Negative RF and anti-CCP antibody assay do not always exclude RA. Patients would require specialist review to exclude the diagnosis.

## What's new?

Starting patients on *disease modifying antirheumatic drugs* (DMARDs) early ensures better treatment outcomes and patient response. Biologic therapies (anti-tumour necrosis factor [anti-TNF]) can be introduced for patients with poor disease control who have severe disease as assessed by a high *disease activity score* (DAS). The tool commonly used in clinical practice is *DAS-28* which is a composite score derived from the number of painful joints, the number of swollen joints, the patient's own global assessment of well-being charted on a visual analogue scale and the level of an inflammatory marker (CRP or ESR) (Figures 11.1 through 11.5).

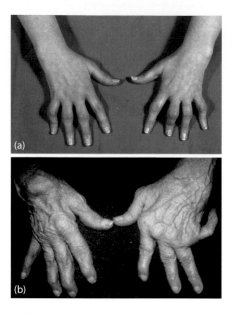

Figure 11.1 **(a)** Proximal interphalangeal involvement in both hands. **(b)** Chronic rheumatoid hand. Note the swan necking deformity of the digits of the right hand and ulnar deviation of the left-hand digits. Both hands show small muscle wasting.

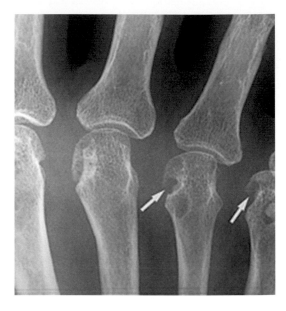

Figure 11.2 Erosions at the periarticular 'bare' areas. These 'bare' areas refer to bone within the synovial space which is not covered by articular cartilage. The marginal 'bare' areas are not covered by cartilage, and the earliest erosions of rheumatoid arthritis are seen here.

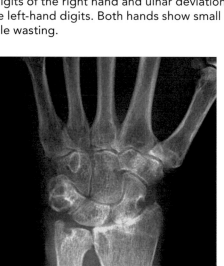

Figure 11.3 Erosive changes at the wrist indicated by red arrows. The wrist is frequently involved in rheumatoid arthritis.

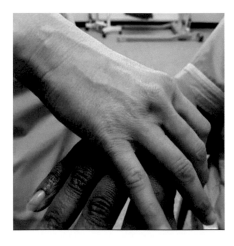

Figure 11.4 Metacarpophalangeal (MCP) joint squeeze in a patient with suspected rheumatoid arthritis (RA). If the patient feels pain this may indicate MCP joint involvement with synovitis.

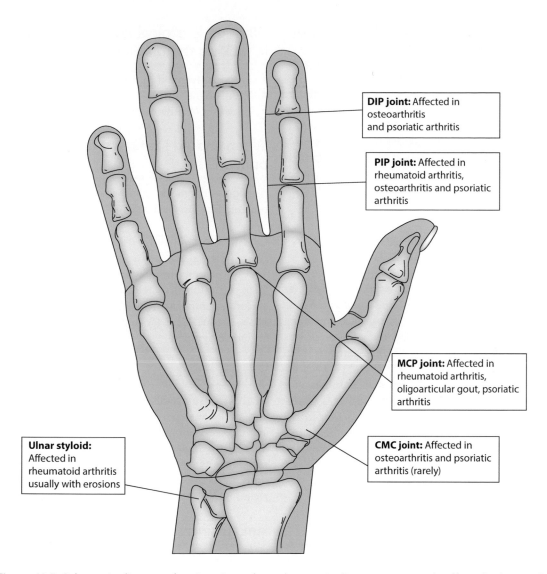

**DIP joint:** Affected in osteoarthritis and psoriatic arthritis

**PIP joint:** Affected in rheumatoid arthritis, osteoarthritis and psoriatic arthritis

**MCP joint:** Affected in rheumatoid arthritis, oligoarticular gout, psoriatic arthritis

**Ulnar styloid:** Affected in rheumatoid arthritis usually with erosions

**CMC joint:** Affected in osteoarthritis and psoriatic arthritis (rarely)

Figure 11.5  Schematic diagram showing sites where rheumatic diseases commonly affect the bone of the hand.

## Seronegative spondyloarthropathies

### Diseases in this group

- Reactive arthritis
- Psoriatic arthritis
- Ankylosing spondylitis (AS)
- Arthritis related to inflammatory bowel disease (formerly called enteropathic arthritis)
- Juvenile spondyloarthropathy

## What is important in the history?

Typically, these conditions display asymmetrical involvement of the large joints, such as knees and ankles which feature strongly. Upper limb joints can also be affected. Specifically ask for peripheral joint pain and swelling. A history of *dactylitis* (inflammation and swelling in one or more digits of the hand or foot) is common in this disease subtype. Patients may also complain of *inflammatory back pain*. This is pain that typically worsens after inactivity and rest, which often improves with exercise and which responds well to non-steroidal anti-inflammatory medication.

Enthesitis such as Achilles tendinopathy, plantar fascitis and medial and lateral epicondylitis tends to occur in this group of patients. *A family history of spondyloarthropathy, positive human leukocyte antigen B-27 test (HLA-B27) and the presence of conditions such as psoriasis, uveitis or inflammatory bowel disease should raise the suspicion for underlying spondyloarthropathy in patients presenting with clinically significant articular symptoms.*

## What focused examination will help to make the diagnosis?

A general examination is undertaken initially (as above) to assess the patient's overall condition. Assess the scalp and skin to check for psoriasis including 'hidden areas' such as behind the ears, umbilicus and natal cleft (when appropriate). It is important to also check for nail pitting. MCP and MTP 'squeeze' may be positive (as above). Entheseal examination is important, checking various entheseal sites (insertion sites of the Achilles' tendon and plantar fascia, medial and lateral epicondyles around the elbow) for tenderness and inflammation. Always assess the sacroiliac joints for tenderness especially in cases where the patient has inflammatory back pain.

## What key investigations should I do?

FBC and inflammatory markers should be checked (see section 'Rheumatoid arthritis'). Check for RF and anti-CCP levels as these markers help to rule out coexistent RA. HLA-B27 assays when positive have prognostic implications but are not used for diagnosis.

X-rays and ultrasound (including entheseal sites) are helpful investigations (see section 'Rheumatoid arthritis').

## How do I manage this condition?

As with RA, patients need early referral to a rheumatologist. NSAIDs can be used whilst patients wait for specialist review. Steroids can be used only after specialist advice but with caution. Note that steroids can make psoriasis worse in cases of psoriatic arthritis.

## What early clinical features will help in making the diagnosis?

- Joint involvement in the presence of psoriasis
- Family history of spondyloarthropathy
- A history of inflammatory bowel disease

## When should I refer for a specialist opinion?

As soon as diagnosis is suspected based on clinical presentation, the specialist opinion should be sought.

## Common pitfalls and how can I avoid these?

Lack of clinically evident synovitis does not exclude spondyloarthropathies as a potential diagnosis. Normal CRP, PV and ESR also do not always exclude diagnosis.

## What's new?

DMARDs are usually commenced in cases where patients have peripheral joint synovitis and symptoms. Biologic therapies can be introduced for select patients with lack of adequate DMARD response. As with RA there are a range of specific tools to assess disease activity that are used by rheumatologists.

## Ankylosing spondylitis

## What is important in the history?

Patients with a history of inflammatory back pain should be evaluated for early AS.

A useful mnemonic here is **I-PAIN**:

I: Insidious onset usually present for >3 months
P: Pain worsens with rest
A: Age of onset <45 years
I: Improves with exercise and NSAID use
N: Night pain that improves on waking up and movement

*Four out of the five above parameters suggest inflammatory back pain.*

Patients may have pain felt deep in the buttocks which may alternate with pain in the lumbar region. This can be a presenting symptom, or the chief complaint. A history of dactylitis and peripheral arthralgia or swelling (suggestive of synovitis) is important. Entheseal involvement is also very common in this group of patients, as is a family history of AS, or the presence of HLA-B27 positivity, psoriasis, uveitis or inflammatory bowel disease.

## What focused examination will help to make the diagnosis?

A general examination is undertaken initially (as above) to assess the patient's overall condition.

Examination of the spine should be undertaken to assess the range of movements in the cervical, thoracic and lumbar regions in the standard planes of flexion, extension, lateral flexion and rotation to ascertain if there is restriction of movement. In addition to global or focal reduction of spinal movements, the following tests are commonly helpful in a clinical setting:

- *Chest expansion*: Chest expansion of less than 2 inches is suggestive of thoracic spine involvement in AS.
- *Schober's test*: Lumbar spine 'opening' during forward flexion of less than 2.5 inches is suggestive of lumbar spine involvement in AS.

Entheseal site examination to check for tenderness should be undertaken. These sites include medial and lateral humeral epicondyles, greater trochanters of the femur, achilles tendon insertion point and the plantar fascia. Sacroiliac joint tenderness and dactylitis are other specific features to look for.

## What key investigations should I do?

FBC and inflammatory markers should be checked (please see earlier sections).

HLA-B27 positivity aids in diagnosis. In Caucasians, 90%–95% of cases of AS are HLA-B27 positive.

X-rays and ultrasound (including entheseal sites) are helpful investigations (please see earlier sections).

## How do I manage this condition?

Patients need early referral to a rheumatologist (as with most rheumatic diseases). NSAIDs are important in reducing inflammation in this condition. Advise the patients to do exercises and stretches whilst they await specialist review, and refer for physiotherapy. There is very little role for steroids in this condition.

## What early clinical features will help in making the diagnosis?

- The presence of symptoms in the patient with a family history of AS
- HLA-B27 positivity
- The coexistence of conditions such as psoriasis, uveitis and inflammatory bowel disease

## Common pitfalls and how can I avoid these?

Failing to obtain a history of inflammatory back pain and other (HLA-B27 related) specific conditions (as above) can lead to diagnostic delay. A negative HLA-B27 test does not exclude diagnosis. Be wary of the patient who has presented on multiple occasions with 'back pain' and who may have normocytic normochromic anaemia on FBC.

## What's new?

Biologic therapies can be introduced in secondary care. There is emerging evidence that the early use of biologics may be particularly helpful in patients with AS. Selection is based on the level of disease activity as assessed by two commonly used clinical measurement tools – the BASDAI (Bath Ankylosing Spondylitis Disease Activity) and BASFI (Bath Ankylosing Spondylitis Functional Index). Traditional DMARDs may be helpful in patients with peripheral synovitis (Figures 11.6 through 11.9).

## Osteoarthritis

## What is important in the history?

Patients complain of pain in the hips, knees or hands (distal interphalangeal joints or base of thumb). Pain in these areas is often worse after effort. Symptoms are usually present continuously for greater than 3 months. Stiffness in the affected joints is usually less than 30 minutes. Check for any history of past trauma which increases likelihood of future OA. Co-existent RA increases the likelihood of patients getting OA. A positive family history of OA may be elicited in patients with nodal OA (FNOA: familial nodal osteoarthritis). Functional disability due to symptoms is prominent in patients with OA.

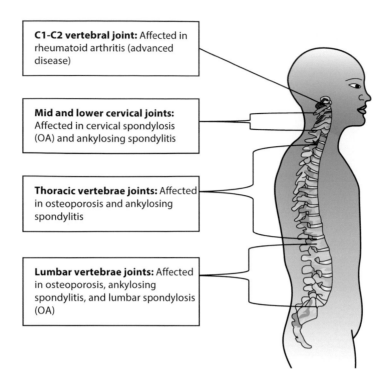

**C1-C2 vertebral joint:** Affected in rheumatoid arthritis (advanced disease)

**Mid and lower cervical joints:** Affected in cervical spondylosis (OA) and ankylosing spondylitis

**Thoracic vertebrae joints:** Affected in osteoporosis and ankylosing spondylitis

**Lumbar vertebrae joints:** Affected in osteoporosis, ankylosing spondylitis, and lumbar spondylosis (OA)

Figure 11.6 Schematic showing the sites in the spinal joints affecting by various rheumatic diseases.

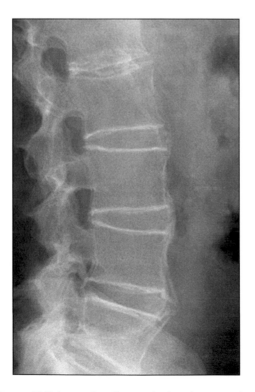

Figure 11.7 Lateral radiograph showing anterior syndesmophytes.

## What focused examination will help to make the diagnosis?

Joint examination should specifically include checking for crepitus and joint line tenderness especially in lower limb joints. Range of movement of affected joints may be reduced. Muscle wasting can be observed around painful joints due to lack of use; for example in prolonged knee OA, thigh muscle wasting may be observed.

## What key investigations should I do?

CRP, PV or ESR are often normal and are helpful in ruling out an inflammatory arthropathy. X-rays are required to assess the degree of damage to affected joints. Signs of OA seen on x-rays include joint space narrowing, osteophyte formation and subchondral sclerosis. Weight-bearing x-ray of the knee reveals better the degree of joint space narrowing.

## How do I manage this condition?

Patient education is paramount with emphasis on the need to keep moving the affected joints

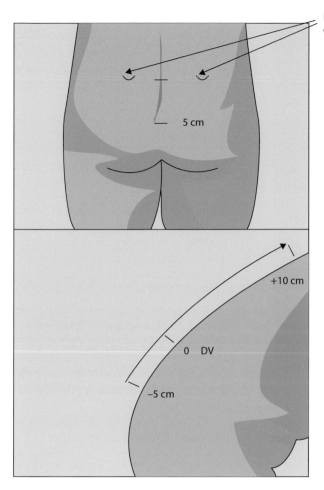

Posterior superior illiac spine
or dimples of Venus **(DV)**

5 cm

+10 cm

0   DV

−5 cm

Figure 11.8 Flexion of lumbar spine measured as increase in distance between points 5 cm below and 10 cm above the level of the dimples of Venus (DV) or posterior superior iliac spine. The finger-floor test is not appropriate, as this mainly tests hip flexion.

and exercising them. Lifestyle advice, exercise and weight loss for foot/ankle OA is also helpful. Topical NSAIDs, starting with paracetamol as the initial therapy then alternative oral analgesia, may be considered.

## What early clinical features will help in making the diagnosis?

- Loss of internal rotation in hip joint OA tends to occur early in the process.
- Hard bony deformities in hand OA – in proximal and distal interphalangeal joints (Bouchard's and Heberden's nodes).

## When should I refer for a specialist opinion?

Generally managed in primary care but refractory cases can be referred for specialist review.

Referral to secondary care is advised in cases refractory to intra-articular injections or when surgical intervention is required.

## Common pitfalls and how can I avoid these?

Wrist, elbow and ankle joints are less commonly affected by OA and if involved may have another underlying cause.

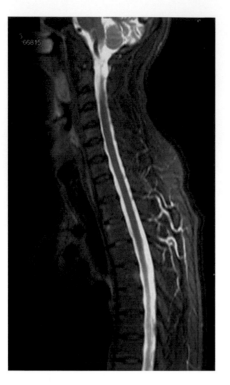

Figure 11.9 Shiny corner or early erosion in ankylosing spondylitis. Early erosions are picked up on magnetic resonance imaging (MRI) scanning.

## What's new?

Self-management with patient education emphasising the importance of exercise and maintaining mobility is key in the overall management of OA (Figure 11.10).

## Septic arthritis

### What is important in the history?

Patients with a short history of a swollen and painful joint (or joints) with restriction of movement should be regarded as having septic arthritis until proven otherwise. A history of systemic features such as fever, malaise is important. Predisposing factors such as diabetes, advanced age, RA, recent joint injection, prosthetic joint and skin infection should be sought.

### What focused examination will help to make the diagnosis?

Joint examination should be undertaken to check for increased warmth, tenderness and reduced range of movement.

Remember that absence of pyrexia in the patient does not exclude the diagnosis.

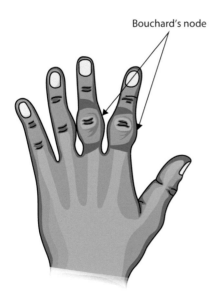
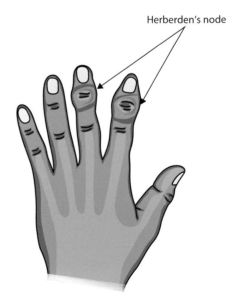

Figure 11.10 Schematic showing the location of Bouchard's and Herberden's node in osteoarthritis of the hand.

## What key investigations should I do?

Inflammatory markers will be elevated but do not wait for blood tests before intervention is sought.

## How do I manage this condition?

Urgent referral to secondary care either under orthopaedics or rheumatology is paramount.

## What early clinical features will help in making the diagnosis?

A history of a painful, swollen single joint is key.

## When should I refer for a specialist opinion?

Urgent referral to secondary care without needing to wait for blood results is indicated.

## Common pitfalls and how can I avoid these?

Absence of fever does not exclude the diagnosis. Always consider the possibility in a patient presenting with a hot swollen single joint.

## What's new?

Joint wash out to dryness in select cases usually done by the orthopaedic team.

# Systemic lupus erythematosus and connective tissue diseases

## What is important in the history?

Due to the multisystem nature of these disease groups, a thorough history is required. Patients may complain of joint pains and swelling which may be migratory or persistent. They may have constitutional symptoms such as fever, night sweats and fatigue. Any history of photosensitive rash, oral or nasal ulcers, Raynaud's phenomenon and serositis suggests an underlying connective tissue disease (CTD). Drug history is important in cases of drug-induced lupus. Patients may also have dry eyes and dry mouth indicative of primary or secondary Sjogren's syndrome.

## What focused examination will help to make the diagnosis?

General examination should be undertaken to assess the patient's overall condition and depending on the presenting complaint(s), a focused examination of the relevant system(s) should be performed.

## What key investigations should I do?

The FBC should be checked, which may show *lymphopaenia as well as anaemia, neutropaenia and thrombocytopenia in certain cases. ESR and PV will often be high. CRP is often normal in SLE despite severe disease.* An elevated CRP in someone with SLE is usually indicative of underlying infection.

*Positive antinuclear antibodies* (ANA) are typically present with titres higher than or equal to 1:160. Antibodies to double-stranded DNA (*anti-DsDNA*) are only positive in 30% of patients with SLE. A urine dipstick assessment should be conducted to exclude the presence of blood and protein, which, if present, suggests an acute nephritic process. This should prompt urgent secondary care referral, and the urea and electrolytes (U&Es) should also be checked.

## How do I manage this condition?

Patients need urgent referral for specialist review once diagnosis is suspected. Do not give steroids unless advised by a specialist. This may reduce symptoms and delay diagnosis in secondary care.

## What early clinical features will help in making the diagnosis?

Patients presenting with joint symptoms may also have the following:

- A photosensitive (malar or front of neck and upper chest) rash
- Raynaud's phenomena
- Recurrent early miscarriage >3 before 10 weeks of gestation or one loss after 10 weeks
- Persistent or 'unexplained' neutropaenia or thrombocytopenia

## When should I refer for a specialist opinion?

There should be a referral to secondary care as soon as diagnosis is suspected. Any evidence of multisystem involvement should also prompt urgent referral.

## Common pitfalls and how can I avoid these?

Consider infection in cases of SLE if CRP is disproportionately high. A positive ANA in isolation does not confirm the diagnosis as normal healthy population may have a positive ANA. Low titre ANA must always be interpreted within the specific clinical context and does not automatically signify underlying SLE.

## What's new?

Once the diagnosis is confirmed DMARDs are usually started. Hydroxychloroquine is often the initial DMARD of choice. Severe cases can be given biologic therapy and immunosuppressive therapy usually commenced in secondary care (Figure 11.11).

## Gout

## What is important in the history?

A history of one or more episodes of monoarticular arthritis followed by intercritical period(s) completely free of symptoms is typical. Maximal symptoms occur within 24–48 hours and are

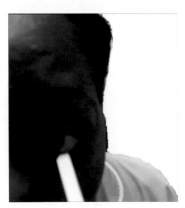

Figure 11.11 Schirmer test with filter paper in the lateral canthus in the left eye. Positive test of less than 5 mm of tear in 5 minutes is highly suggestive of dry eye–related sicca symptoms.

usually evident from the history. Some patients have a history of unilateral first metatarsophalangeal joint attack (podagra) either as a first presentation or recurrent episodes. A history of predisposing factors such as family history, high alcohol use, use of diuretics, undertreated hypothyroidism and diet rich in purines and fructose-containing drinks need to be explored.

## What focused examination will help to make the diagnosis?

Joint examination to check for increased warmth, tenderness and reduced range of movement in the affected joint or joints is essential.

## What key investigations should I do?

Inflammatory markers such as CRP are typically elevated in the acute phase. Urate levels are usually high but may be normal during an acute attack. Urate levels tend to be high during the intercritical period. X-rays are important if tophi are present to determine whether there may be bony involvement.

## How do I manage this condition?

NSAIDs or colchicine should be introduced early once gout is suspected. Predisposing factors should also be addressed such as alcohol reduction, weight loss and consideration of diuretic therapy alteration. Also lifestyle modification is important.

Oral steroids can be used at around a dose of 30 mg for 1 week of prednisolone for cases with impaired renal function or intolerance of colchicine or NSAIDs.

If there are more than two attacks a year, then usually allopurinol is the drug of choice to lower the urate level should be commenced ideally >2 weeks from an acute attack. The patient should have NSAID/colchicine cover when allopurinol is started and again with each dose increase.

## What early clinical features will help in making the diagnosis?

- A typical history with podagra
- Recurrent short episodes of inflammation affecting just one or a few joints
- The presence of predisposing factors

## When should I refer for a specialist opinion?

Patients with refractory symptoms that do not settle with conventional treatment should be referred to see a specialist.

## Common pitfalls and how can I avoid these?

A normal urate level does not exclude gout.

## What's new?

'Treat to target' in gout: the aim of therapy is to get the urate level below 360 nmol/L in non-tophaceous gout and less than 300 nmol/L in tophaceous gout. Febuxostat can be started in patients who may have an allergy to allopurinol or if allopurinol is not effective in maximum tolerated doses (Figure 11.12).

## Polymyalgia rheumatica and giant cell arteritis

## What is important in the history?

A history of new headache usually in the temporal region, or occasionally in the occipital region,

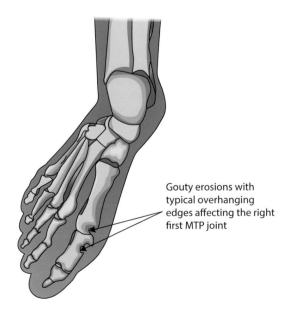

Gouty erosions with typical overhanging edges affecting the right first MTP joint

Figure 11.12 Schematic showing gouty arthritis with erosions in the right first metatarsophalangeal (MTP) joint.

in someone over the age of 55 years, should prompt the consideration of giant cell arteritis (GCA). Patients with polymyalgia rheumatica (PMR) usually present with stiffness (more than pain) in the shoulders and hip that comes on over a few days or weeks. If headaches are present in a patient with PMR then GCA must be considered and excluded. Patients may have constitutional symptoms such as fever, night sweats and fatigue and weight loss in cases of PMR and GCA. Ask about jaw claudication, visual disturbance such as diplopia, transient (or permanent) visual loss. There may be a history of scalp pain as well in GCA.

## What focused examination will help to make the diagnosis?

Check for temporal artery signs such as differences in appearance, pulse intensity and tenderness along artery. Systolic blood pressure differences in both arms of the patient greater than 20 mmHg are regarded as significant.

## What key investigations should I do?

Inflammatory markers such as CRP, PV and ESR nearly always elevated. Anaemia and reactive thrombocytosis may be seen.

## How do I manage this condition?

In cases of suspected GCA with headaches and raised inflammatory markers, start steroids and refer to secondary care. In cases of suspected GCA without raised inflammatory markers, seek specialist advice as another diagnosis is highly likely. The dose of steroids depends on the symptoms present. With the presence of visual symptoms or jaw claudication, the patient should receive prednisolone 60 mg immediately and then daily until specialist review.

In the absence of jaw claudication and visual symptoms, prescribe prednisolone 40 mg daily for 3 weeks then taper down until specialist review. PMR is usually treated with no more than 15 mg of prednisolone daily. Lack of response to 15 mg of prednisolone suggests the diagnosis is in doubt.

## What early clinical features will help in making the diagnosis?

- The presence of early constitutional symptoms with a history suggestive of PMR or GCA
- A history of stiffness in shoulder or pelvic muscles that may progress to a maximum intensity usually in a few days to a few weeks

## When should I refer for a specialist opinion?

Referral to a specialist is recommended early in GCA. It is pertinent to note that PMR is generally managed in primary care.

## Common pitfalls and how can I avoid these?

GCA and PMR are rarely ever diagnosed in patients under the age of 50 years. Steroids must be tapered very slowly once commenced in cases confirmed by a rheumatologist. Patients with GCA or PMR usually require treatment for between 1 and 2 years.

## What's new?

Early use of DMARDs now occurs in patients with GCA and PMR, especially if the patient after a year or 18 months isn't able to wean off prednisolone. Patients on long-term steroids will need concurrent medications such as proton pump inhibitors, calcium and vitamin D, and a bisphosphonate.

## Systemic vasculitis

## What is important in the history?

Patients complain of joint pains and swelling which may be migratory or persistent. They may have constitutional symptoms such as fever, night sweats and fatigue. A non-blanching skin rash may be present. Other features in the history may include epistaxis, haemoptysis, Raynaud's phenomenon and limb paraesthesia. Drug history is important as certain drug allergies may mimic vasculitis.

## What focused examination will help to make the diagnosis?

A general examination must be undertaken to assess the patient's overall condition, and depending on the presenting complaint examine the relevant system. Look specifically for signs of cutaneous vasculitis (non-blanching rash over the legs), nail fold infarcts and palatal or scleral haemorrhages. Check for pedal oedema and any respiratory signs.

## What key investigations should I do?

FBC may show anaemia and thrombocytopenia in certain cases. Inflammatory markers will often be elevated. ANA and anti-neutrophilic cytoplasmic antibodies (ANCA) can be requested whilst the patient is awaiting specialist review. Urine dipstick assessment is required to exclude the presence of blood and protein. If present, this suggests an acute nephritic process. A full biochemical profile should be requested which includes U&Es, liver enzymes and bone profile.

## How do I manage this condition?

Patients require urgent referral for specialist review once diagnosis is suspected. Do not give steroids unless advised by a rheumatologist. This may dampen symptoms and delay definitive diagnosis in secondary care.

## What early clinical features will help in making the diagnosis?

- The presence of polyarthralgia with non-blanching skin rash
- Multisystem involvement
- Fatigue and low energy levels

## When should I refer for a specialist opinion?

Urgent review by a rheumatologist is required as soon as the diagnosis is suspected.

## Common pitfalls and how can I avoid these?

Normal FBC and inflammatory markers do not rule out the diagnosis. A positive ANCA does not always confirm diagnosis but can be highly suggestive of the diagnosis. ANCA levels are helpful in monitoring disease activity.

## What's new?

Once the diagnosis is confirmed in secondary care then steroids and DMARDs are commenced early.

In severe case or life-threatening situations, immunosuppressive drugs or biologic therapy are other therapeutic options.

## Fibromyalgia

## What is important in the history?

Patients may complain of joint pains but there is usually an absence of joint swelling despite pain. A history of generalised widespread pain without constitutional symptoms is typical. Patients also have poor non-restorative sleep and fatigue. They also have difficulty coping with activities of daily living.

## What focused examination will help to make the diagnosis?

Check for tender 'fibromyalgia' points. These 18 points are located at the back of the cervical spine, between the shoulder blades and around the shoulders and trochanteric bursa. Fibromyalgia is

---

### SUMMARY

In this chapter, we have considered rheumatological conditions that are commonly seen in general practice. We have provided key clinical features in a practical format that might assist a busy GP in recognising or diagnosing these conditions, as well as instituting an initial management plan.

Rheumatology covers a wide range of conditions and the authors are mindful that in an emerging era of increasing complexity in general practice the primary care clinician cannot be expected to know 'everything about rheumatology'. The 'take home message' that they would like to leave for the reader is simply expressed as follows: if in doubt ask for specialist rheumatology advice.

---

diagnosed if there are 11 or more positive points. Physical examination is usually normal, and there is a striking absence of joint swelling or inflammation despite joint pains.

## What key investigations should I do?

FBC, urea and electrolytes and inflammatory markers such as CRP, PV and ESR are almost always normal. Check for vitamin D deficiency which can cause generalised widespread pain. It is important to also evaluate the creatine kinase (CK) levels.

## How do I manage this condition?

Patients need advice on a graded exercise regime once diagnosis is confirmed, as this ensures long-term favourable outcomes. Simple analgesia and use of anti-neuropathic medication as adjuncts can be helpful.

## What early clinical features will help in making the diagnosis?

- Poor non-restorative sleep
- Generalised widespread pain
- Normal blood results
- Long standing history
- Depression

## When should I refer for a specialist opinion?

Cases where there is diagnostic uncertainty should be referred to a rheumatologist.

## Common pitfalls and how can I avoid these?

Diagnosing fibromyalgia in the presence of unexplained abnormal blood results should be with caution. Always check for vitamin D levels and thyroid function.

## What's new?

Firm reassurance with an emphasis on patient self-management concerning graded exercise regimes and lifestyle modification is the mainstay of treatment.

## Acknowledgement

The authors are grateful to Dr. Lisa Neville for reviewing this chapter and providing helpful comments from a primary care perspective.

## References

1. Al-Sukaini A, Azam M, Samanta A. *Rheumatology: A Clinical Handbook.* Banbury, UK: Scion Publishing Limited, 2014.

2. Petri M, Orbai AM, Alarcón GS, Gordon C, Merrill JT, Fortin PR et al. Derivation and validation of the Systemic Lupus International Collaborating Clinics classification criteria for systemic lupus erythematosus. *Arthritis Rheum.* 2012;64:2677.

3. Sieper J, van der Heijde D, Landewé R, Brandt J, Burgos-Vagas R, Collantes-Estevez E et al. New criteria for inflammatory back pain in patients with chronicback pain: A real patient exercise by experts from the Assessment of Spondyloarthritis International Society (ASAS). *Ann Rheum Dis.* 2009;68:784.

4. Watts RA, Scott DG. Recent developments in the classification and assessment of vasculitis. *Best Pract Res Clin Rheumatol.* 2009;23:429.

5. Aletaha D, Neogi T, Silman AJ, Funovits J, Felson DT, Bingham CO 3rd et al. Rheumatoid arthritis classification criteria: An American College of Rheumatology/European League Against Rheumatism collaborative initiative. *Arthritis Rheum.* 2010;62:2569.

# 12

# The role of physiotherapy for musculoskeletal disorders in primary care

RICHARD WOOD

## Introduction

Musculoskeletal (MSK) physiotherapists provide expert assessment, diagnosis and treatment planning for patients with MSK pain and dysfunction. They have amalgamated detailed anatomical, physiological and pathological knowledge to provide a broad range of skills across primary and secondary care. They are in a unique position to bridge that important interface. In turn, this provides clinically efficient and cost-effective services across the health-care community.[1]

A physiotherapist's core skills include exercise prescription, manual therapy, graded rehabilitation and promotion of self-management. These core skills improve independence, enable improved function and ultimately lead to a variety of health gains in individuals. This chapter concentrates on a list of commonly seen MSK conditions in primary care. In any 1 year, 20% of the general practitioner (GP) registered population may consult their GP with an MSK problem. In those aged over 50, this may be as high as 30%. It is generally accepted that about 30% of GP consultations are for MSK conditions.[2] It is a very common cause of repeat consultations.

This chapter highlights the key areas of examination and management strategies including simple exercise prescription. There is also a suggestion of when to refer to an MSK triage service or orthopaedic consultant. The conditions are discussed in no particular order but from the author's experience are very relevant to conditions likely to be seen.

Each of the following sections will give a brief history, and outline key examination features, management/rehabilitation strategies and when to refer guidelines. There are pictures of stretches and strengthening exercises at the end of the chapter. A list of 'not to miss problems' are also included.

## Anterior knee pain

Anterior knee pain can affect any age but is common in adolescents. It is estimated that around 25% of exercising adolescents will develop anterior knee pain. There is usually no history of trauma. The pain is located to the front of the knee joint and aggravated by descending stairs and squatting. It can cause pseudolocking of the joint. It is not unusual for older patients to present with isolated patellofemoral osteoarthritis (OA).

### KEY EXAMINATION FEATURES

- No joint line tenderness
- Pain on compression of the patellofemoral joint
- Tight hamstrings
- Tight gastrocnemius
- Weak quadriceps
- Poor single leg stability
- Exclude hip pathology (ensure good flexion, abduction and medial rotation)

## Management strategy

It is very important to give a clear explanation of the disorder and useful to explain the difference between the patellofemoral joint and the tibiofemoral joint. Describing the knee to patients in terms of compartments is extremely useful. Patients often find this type of problem frustrating, particularly exercising individuals. Activity modification (finding alternative exercise) and avoiding aggravating activity is very useful.

## Rehabilitation

- Advice regarding stretching hamstrings (refer to exercises at the end of the chapter, Figure 12.2)
- Advice regarding calf stretching (Figure 12.3)
- Simple quad strengthening (Figures 12.4 and 12.5)

## When to refer?

Patients with anterior knee pain can usually be managed in primary care but if they are not improving then formal referral to physiotherapy should be considered. If there is concern over the diagnosis or if the patient is a high demand athlete, then an early referral is advised. Patients who have a history of 'mechanical' symptoms, i.e. recurrent subluxations or frank dislocations, should also have a timely referral for specialist assessment.

## Medial knee joint pain (degenerative medial meniscus/medial OA flare)

This is a common complaint in patients in the fifth and sixth decades of life. There is usually no history of significant trauma associated with the onset. The pain is usually specific to the medial aspect of the knee joint. There can be an effusion but usually no mechanical features of giving way or locking. Clinically differentiating between a degenerative medial meniscus and early OA of the medial compartment can be difficult. Varus alignment with previous history of meniscal surgery can be a clue towards a diagnosis of OA. There is usually weight-bearing pain, pain ascending stairs, night pain and possible loss of movement.

---

### KEY EXAMINATION FEATURES

- Patient may limp
- Tenderness of the medial joint line
- May have loss of terminal extension and flexion
- Weakness of quadriceps and gastrocnemius
- Effusion in joint (possible)
- Exclude hip pathology (ensure good flexion, abduction and medial rotation)

---

## Management strategy

As with previous management, a clear explanation is very important. The prognosis for this type of problem in the absence of mechanical symptoms is very good with most symptoms settling in 6–8 weeks. Simple remedies in the acute stage with ice, rest and activity modification are appropriate.

## Rehabilitation

- Quadriceps strengthening (Figures 12.4 and 12.5)
- Gastrocnemius strengthening (Figure 12.3)
- Gluteal strengthening (Figure 12.6)

## When to refer?

It can be useful to refer patients who are not improving over 8–12 weeks (although some may settle beyond this time). If patients develop 'mechanical' symptoms on a regular basis, then referral to orthopaedics or for a magnetic resonance imaging (MRI) may be indicated. It is useful to refer patients earlier if they have had previous surgery or if they have varus alignment of the knee.

## Patella tendinopathy

Patella tendinopathy can present in many age groups and is usually found in active individuals. There is no trauma related to this condition and it is largely caused by overuse. Identification of factors such as activity level/type, footwear, weight, loading capacity and biomechanics are key considerations. The pain is usually located specifically at the inferior pole of the patella tendon, which is tender to palpate. Descending stairs and pain when loading are aggravating factors.

---

### KEY EXAMINATION FEATURES

- Good range of movement
- Specific tenderness at the inferior pole of patella at tendon–bone junction
- May have tight hamstrings and calf muscles
- May have poor stability when standing on affected leg indicating quadriceps and gluteal weakness

---

## Management strategy

This can be a challenging problem to deal with, as often it will take many months to improve, so managing the expectation of the patient is paramount. It can be useful to advise activity modification (but not complete rest) in the early stages to promote recovery. Often prolonged progressive rehabilitation (eccentric loading) is required and anecdotally early referral to physiotherapy is appropriate.

## Rehabilitation

- Hamstring stretch (Figure 12.2)
- Gastrocnemius stretch (Figure 12.3)
- Quadriceps strengthening (Figures 12.4 and 12.5) – useful in acute phase
- Gastrocnemius strengthening (Figure 12.7)

## When to refer?

As already stated, active individuals will find this problem particularly frustrating, and early referral for formal physiotherapy may be appropriate. In some cases, it may take 4–6 months to improve. It is not necessary to consider imaging if the clinical diagnosis is certain. If patients fail to improve then onward referral for consideration of *shock-wave therapy* may be considered. Surgery can be considered but is rarely required.

## Shoulder impingement

Shoulder impingement usually presents insidiously over time without trauma. Patients with acute non-traumatic shoulder pain with a loss of movement should be investigated for calcific tendinopathy (x-ray to confirm diagnosis) or septic arthritis (urgent bloods and referral). The pain is usually located to the shoulder joint but can be specific to the anterior aspect. Pain can be referred to the elbow. Patients will describe a catching pain specific to movement and possible night pain when lying on the affected side. Shoulder impingement will usually not give neurological symptoms in the affected arm.

---

### KEY EXAMINATION FEATURES

- Patients will have a good range of movement.
- Patients are likely to have poor posture (thoracic kyphosis and forward head posture).
- May demonstrate an abduction arc of pain.
- The rotator cuff power is good.
- May have a positive Hawkins and Kennedy test, empty can test, full can test or Neer test (the sensitivity and specificity of specific shoulder tests are generally poor).
- Exclude cervical radiculopathy by asking patient to rotate cervical spine to the affected side, combined with side flexion to the affected side. (Be suspicious of cervical involvement if shoulder or arm discomfort is reproduced with this movement.)

## Management strategy

A clear explanation to alleviate patient's concerns is very helpful as patients are often anxious about 'tears' and 'frozen shoulders'. It is useful to give simple postural advice to limit thoracic flexion and forward head posture. If there are concerns in relation to work position, then advice about ergonomic assessment is appropriate. If pain is an ongoing significant feature, then consideration of a subacromial injection is worthwhile adjunct to physiotherapy.

## Rehabilitation

- Strengthen shoulder extensors and lateral rotators (Figures 12.8 and 12.9)
- Strengthen scapular retractors and thoracic extensors (pull shoulders backwards)

## When to refer?

Patients who do not improve over a 3–4 month period and who have had suggested treatment strategies can be considered for onward referral.

It is generally acceptable to try two subacromial injections in this time period. If patients appear to have complex, dysfunctional movement patterns of the shoulder and scapula then early referral to physiotherapy should be considered.

An ultrasound scan is not required unless there is significant movement loss with a history of trauma which would suggest a large rotator cuff tear.

## Shoulder capsulitis: 'frozen shoulder'

A frozen shoulder can present secondary to OA (slow onset), minor trauma (fast onset) or idiopathically (slow or fast onset). There is an association with ischaemic heart disease, diabetes and smoking. Typically, there are three phases, 'freezing', 'frozen' and 'thawing'. Patients may present in any of these phases. Patients will have non-specific shoulder pain, night pain and importantly a restriction of active and passive movement. It is unusual for paediatric, adolescent and young adults to present with a frozen shoulder and a differential diagnosis should be considered.

---

### KEY EXAMINATION FEATURES

- Pain and restriction of movement in the capsular pattern.
- A typical capsular pattern normally presents with lateral rotation restricted the most, then abduction, then medial rotation (hand behind back).
- There will be a hard end feel to active and passive movement.
- Rotator cuff strength testing will be normal.

---

## Management strategy

Patients who have a 'frozen shoulder' should be counselled from the early stages. Even with treatment, symptoms can last for 24–36 months. In the acute phase, an intra-articular injection adjunct to range of movement exercise may be helpful. This often needs to be parallel to good pain control.

## Rehabilitation

- Simple passive flexion, abduction and lateral rotation are useful (Figure 12.11)
- General functional exercise

## When to refer?

'Frozen' shoulder can be a challenge to treat by any clinician. If the acute pain subsides in 6–8 weeks, then referral to physiotherapy should be the first point of contact to mobilise the shoulder. If pain and stiffness remain (after 8 weeks and an injection has not helped), then referral to an orthopaedic shoulder clinic is advised to explore other options which may include distension arthrograms or manipulation under anaesthesia (MUA).

## Rotator cuff tear

Rotator cuff tears are common without trauma in the sixth and seventh decades of life and may not always be symptomatic in terms of pain or movement loss. Ultrasound scans of entirely asymptomatic shoulders can show complete tendon tears which are often incidental findings. Rotator cuff tears can occur with minor or significant trauma. The main features are usually (1) direct impact onto shoulder and (2) a loss of active movement. The passive range is usually well preserved. Rotator cuff tears under the age of 40 are uncommon; therefore, active movement loss in this age group requires further evaluation.

---

### KEY EXAMINATION FEATURES

- Loss of active movement usually abduction and lateral rotation
- Preserved passive movement
- Loss of power to abduct and externally rotate
- Always consider a possible neural cause in young patients with no associated trauma (e.g. long thoracic nerve palsy or neuralgic amyotrophy)

---

## Management strategy

Identifying this disorder at an early stage is vitally important and should not be confused with a frozen shoulder. Early assessment and further review 2–3/52 after onset are advisable (often patients are too painful to make accurate diagnosis in the early stages). If patients improve over time with good function and diminishing pain, then no further action is required.

## Rehabilitation

- Encourage active and active-assisted movements in the acute phase (Figures 12.11, 12.12 and 12.13)

## When to refer?

Some patients who have large rotator cuff tears will improve functionally (albeit with some pain) over time. However, if younger patients do not improve within 2–3 weeks and have significant movement loss (<90° abduction) then early referral for an ultrasound scan and orthopaedic opinion is necessary. Patients who are over 75 years old are unlikely to be considered for surgery and therefore should be referred to physiotherapy to improve general function.

## Lateral epicondylitis (tennis elbow)

This is one of the most common conditions seen in general practice. The patient presents with pain maximal over the lateral elbow, with some referral into the forearm. It often starts insidiously, but can have a sudden onset. Activities of the forearm and wrist, such as gripping, twisting and extension aggravate symptoms, especially in the 'palm down' position. It does not always occur in tennis players of course, but this description gives a clue to the importance of identifying causative factors such as overuse, training errors, poor technique (backhand) and ergonomic factors at work, for example. A few minutes spent here is well worthwhile, saving time later on management.

---

### KEY EXAMINATION FEATURES

- Always exclude referred pain from the cervical spine/shoulder
- Full range of all passive movements (compare both sides)
- Pain on passive wrist flexion (with elbow extended)
- Resisted tests positive – wrist/middle finger contraction against resistance with the elbow in extension (common extensor tendon/extensor carpi radialis brevis [ECRB] insertion)
- Palpation – tenderness over the anterior facet of the lateral epicondyle, which is best felt with the forearm supinated

It is important to note that the site of this lesion is over the anterior facet of the epicondyle, not its lateral prominence. This is a common misunderstanding, and important for the correct siting of injections (this also reduces risk of steroid atrophy).

---

## Management

This is often a self-limiting condition over a 12-month period. A full explanation and advice on how to address causative factors are paramount. Simple analgesia, topical/oral non-steroidal anti-inflammatory drugs (NSAIDs) may help but do little to address pathology. It can be worthwhile considering a local steroid injection if in significant pain but not as an isolated treatment. Tennis elbow splints appear to help some individuals. Appropriate rehabilitation is the mainstay of treatment.

## Rehabilitation

- Initially simple icing, stretching and static wrist extension exercises (Figures 12.14, and 12.15)
- Progress to eccentric exercise including pronation and supination (Figure 12.16)

## When to refer?

If there is concern over the diagnosis or failure to make improvements over 12 weeks then referral for formal physiotherapy can be helpful. Beyond this surgical treatment, novel treatments such as *autologous blood injections* or *extracorporeal shock-wave therapy* are often considered.

## Olecranon bursa

This is swelling over the posterior elbow. It often presents acutely and can alarm patients, but is easily managed in general practice. It can be caused by direct trauma but is more often due to chronic pressure – e.g. desks, armrests or driving. There can be an inflammatory component, and gout is a rare cause. They can become infected – early oral antibiotics are usually effective.

## Management (almost always conservative)

It is important to avoid all pressure on this area. It usually resolves but can take several weeks. Aspiration can be considered for resistant cases but consider the risk of infection and persisting sinus with discharge. This often recurs if the pressure factors are not addressed. Surgery is a last resort and rarely necessary and often leaves residual sensitivity.

In practice, it can be useful to aspirate the acute traumatic (haemorrhagic) ones, but otherwise treat conservatively advising avoidance of pressure.

## Distal biceps insertion rupture

This is worth a mention, since although rare, it is important not to miss – delay in diagnosis and treatment can have a significant long-term effect on function.

In comparison to long head of biceps rupture (proximal origin), patients are usually younger and present with an acute severe 'strain' after heavy lifting or similar. Pain swelling and bruising are often prominent. Tenderness is a feature, but can be difficult to localise specifically at the site of biceps insertion because of swelling. Resisted elbow flexion and supination (more sensitive) are weak and painful. If suspected, urgent orthopaedic review is required.

## Proximal biceps rupture

Although this problem can look quite dramatic (*Popeye deformity*) and concerning for a patient, no urgent action needs to be taken unlike a distal biceps rupture (see above). Patients tend to be older and have a history of trauma. They will often experience a 'pop' and often bruise. This rarely causes any functional difficulty and is not amenable to surgical intervention. Patients require accurate assessment and an explanation of the disorder. Most patients will not require any onward referral unless function is a problem and a physiotherapy referral may be helpful.

## Achilles tendinopathy

This condition can affect active and non-active individuals. It can be debilitating and take months to improve even with early expert treatment. It is important to establish what has contributed to the onset of the problem for future management. Most patients will prevent with mid-portion tendon pain and swelling which is tender to palpate. Early activity modification, relative rest, icing and non-steroidals are appropriate initially.

### KEY EXAMINATION FEATURES

- Usually unilateral
- Local tenderness 6–8 cm from insertion point on calcaneum
- May have swelling/thickening
- Patient may limp at onset

## Management strategy

In active individuals, the importance of long-term outcome with graded rehabilitation is worthwhile to explain. There is no quick fix for Achilles tendon pain. It is not uncommon for problems to persist for 3–6 months. Activity modification and icing should start immediately after the problem is identified. An early referral to physiotherapy is usually advised.

## Rehabilitation

- Gastrocnemius stretch (Figure 12.3)
- Static gastrocnemius strengthening (Figure 12.7) – useful in early stages
- Eccentric gastrocnemius and soleus exercise can be useful at the right stage of rehabilitation

## When to refer?

An early referral to physiotherapy is recommended after the diagnosis is made. Often 3 months of careful treatment is required. If patients fail to progress, then onward referral for consideration of *shock-wave therapy* can be considered. Surgical treatment is sometimes considered.

## Plantar fasciitis

Plantar fasciitis presents acutely or can be of insidious onset. Often a change of activity, footwear and weight gain can be a contributing factor. Pain is the predominant feature and in 80% of cases located to the anteromedial portion of the calcaneus where the plantar fascia inserts. The pain is usually worse first thing in the morning and after periods of rest. The pain will often improve with light activity as the 'start-up' pain subsides.

---

### KEY EXAMINATION FEATURES

- The patient may limp.
- Usually localised pain to the anteromedial calcaneum.
- Should be tender in the aforementioned area. If not consider differential diagnosis, e.g. fat pad irritation, insertional Achilles. tendinopathy, plantar fibromatosis.
- May have tight hamstrings, gastrocnemius, soleus and long toe flexors.
- The plantar fascia may also be tight.
- The patient may have a supinated or pronated foot type.

---

## Management strategy

A clear explanation should be given. Simple measures including gel heel pads, activity modification, ice rolling and massage in the early stages can be helpful. In severe cases, a local steroid injection can be considered. If foot biomechanics are considered to be a contributing factor then referral to podiatry can be considered.

## Rehabilitation

- Stretch hamstrings, calf, toe flexors and plantar fascia (Figures 12.2, 12.3 and 12.17)
- Soft tissue massage to area

## When to refer?

If there is concern over the specific diagnosis or failure to improve over 12 weeks, then further advice and exercise prescription/progression may be required via physiotherapy. Consideration of adjunct therapies such as *shock-wave therapy* or *autologous blood injection* is also useful.

## Mechanical neck pain

This can develop insidiously or with minor trauma. It will lead to pain and neck stiffness. The pain will be located to the neck and upper shoulder region, usually with no referral to the arm. Paraesthesia and anaesthesia would be uncommon with mechanical neck pain. Headaches are common. It is important to exclude any red flags (dizziness, diplopia, drop attacks, dysphagia, dysarthria, tongue numbness, facial numbness, distal symptoms in legs), in addition to usual special questions.

---

### KEY EXAMINATION FEATURES

- Usually unilateral pain
- Cervical rotation and side flexion usually limited
- Poor posture
- Tenderness of paraspinal muscles

---

## Management strategy

It is important to exclude any serious cases and alleviate any fears that the patient may have. Appropriate pain relief/muscle relaxants may be required. Heat packs are extremely useful in the acute phase. Postural and ergonomic advice should be given.

## Rehabilitation

- Gentle range of movement exercise usually best done in supine. Simple rotation exercises work well (Figures 12.8 and 12.19).

## When to refer?

If patients are not functioning well at 6 weeks despite advice and exercise then referral to physiotherapy may be helpful. Patients who have recurrent problems that have benefitted from physiotherapy previously can be referred at an early stage. An onward referral in the absence of concerning pathology is not usually required.

## Mechanical low-back pain

This can be acute or chronic in nature. It is extremely common. Pain can be located to either side of the spine or buttock. It can be extreme and debilitating at onset. Red flags must be excluded for serious spinal pathology. Movement patterns are often distorted in the acute phase. As well as meeting the physical needs of patients in the acute phase, psychological support and counselling are very important.

### KEY EXAMINATION FEATURES

- Exclude neurological signs.
- Exclude red flags and non-MSK causes in acute phase.
- Loss of flexion or extension.
- Often patient is side flexed to left or right and in spasm.
- Ensure hip movements are full and pain free.

## Management strategy

Mechanical low-back pain can be challenging in some individuals. The first interaction with the patient is vitally important. A good explanation to alleviate patient fears is always necessary. Simple pain relief will be required in the acute phase. It can be useful to advise heat/ice depending on patient preference. Advice to remain active within the comfort zone should be encouraged.

## Rehabilitation

- Simple exercise in supine, knee rolling, knees to chest (Figures 12.21, 12.22 and 12.23)

## When to refer to physiotherapy?

Mechanical low-back pain continues to be a very common and challenging problem. If there is no improvement at 6 weeks, then referral to physiotherapy is advised. If there have been multiple acute or chronic episodes of pain, then referral to physiotherapy may be helpful. An onward referral in the absence of concerning pathology is not usually required.

## Low-back pain with radiculopathy

This usually presents with acute onset due to minor trauma, poor lifting or sustained flexed body position. Patients may have a combination of back pain, unilateral leg pain, anaesthesia, paraesthesia and loss of motor power more common in distal muscle groups. Red flags for serious spinal pathology must be excluded. Pain may be worse with spinal flexion or extension with referral to appropriate dermatome. Symptoms may be worse first thing in the morning.

### KEY EXAMINATION FEATURES

- Movement loss usually flexion more than extension but can be varied
- Accurate neurological assessment required and documented (straight leg raise [SLR], reflex, motor, sensory [RMS] testing)
- May have unilateral reduction in SLR
- May have diminished reflex sensation and power related to affected nerve root

## Management strategy

In this situation, a clear explanation of the disorder and prognosis (50% of patients will improve at 6 weeks and 75% at 12 weeks) should be given. It is always important to explain warning signs of cauda equina syndrome and document this. Appropriate pain relief and muscle relaxants in the acute phase are necessary and nerve modifying medication if limb symptoms are ongoing. It is important to monitor neurological signs over time (Figure 12.1).

## Rehabilitation

- Simple exercise in supine, knee rolling, knee to chest. Encourage walking and activity as tolerated. (Figures 12.21, 12.22 and 12.23).

## When to refer?

If there is a suspicion of red flag pathology, refer urgently to an orthopaedic spine clinic or emergency department especially if you suspect cauda equina syndrome. If symptoms are stable but there is poor function, then referral to physiotherapy is advised.

## Not-to-miss MSK disorders: if suspected there should be immediate referral to secondary care specialist service

- Cauda equina syndrome
- Suspicion of metastatic cord compression
- Acute limb neurological deficit
- Suspicion of progressive cervical myelopathy
- Suspicion of a septic joint
- Distal biceps rupture
- Suspicion of a subscapularis rupture
- Suspicion of patella tendon/quadriceps tendon rupture
- Suspicion of Achilles tendon rupture
- Suspicion of a femoral neck stress fracture
- Suspicion of bone tumour or metastatic bone pain
- Suspected scaphoid fracture in a young person

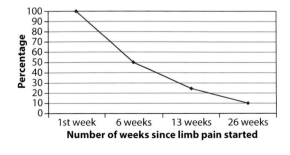

Figure 12.1 Number of patients who are complaining of nerve root pain over time.

## Exercises

1. Hamstring stretch 10 × 10/15 second hold × 2 day (Figure 12.2).
2. Calf stretch 10 × 10/15 second hold × 2/day (Figure 12.3).
3. Static wall squat 3 × 1 minute hold × 2/day (must be pain free) (Figures 12.4 and 12.5).
4. Standing at wall, bend knee and lift leg backwards to strengthen gluteal muscles, hold for 5 seconds and repeat × 20 (Figure 12.6).
5. Calf raise – stand on one leg and push up on toes then drop down. 2 × 20 raises × 2/day (Figure 12.7).
6. Pull elbow back and twist arm out, hold for 2 seconds, repeat movement × 10 and do × 2 sets × 2/day (Figure 12.8).

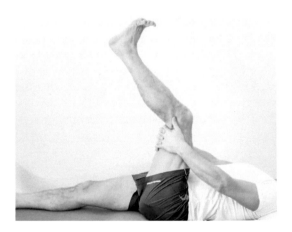

Figure 12.2 Hamstring stretch.

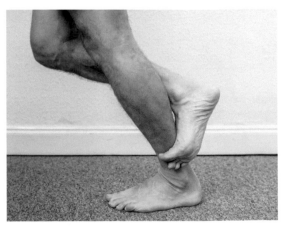

Figure 12.3 Calf stretch.

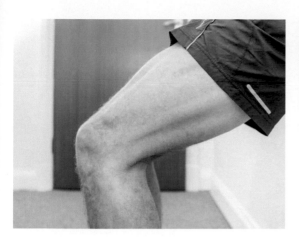

Figure 12.4  Quadriceps strengthening.

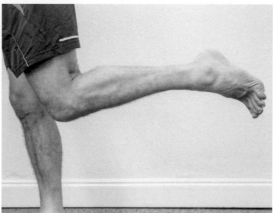

Figure 12.6  Gluteal strengthening.

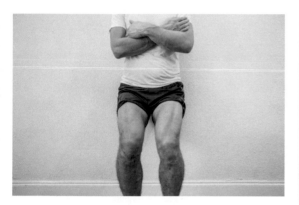

Figure 12.5  Quadriceps strengthening.

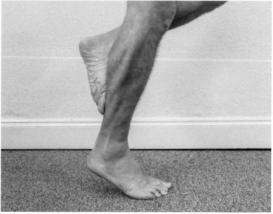

Figure 12.7  Calf strengthening.

7. Pull both elbows backwards and stick chest out, hold for 2 seconds, repeat movement × 10 and do × 2 sets × 2/day (Figure 12.9).
8. Practice walking up and down wall with both hands, aim to do × 20 with each arm (Figure 12.10).
9. Stretch capsule 10 × 10 second hold × 2 × 2/day (Figure 12.11).
10. Practice lifting arm up and out with back against wall × 10 × 2/day (hold for 2 seconds at limit) (Figure 12.12).
11. Twist arm out with back against wall × 10 × 2/day (hold for 2 seconds at limit) (Figure 12.13).
12. Stretch arm downwards and hold for 15 seconds, repeat × 10 × 2/day (Figure 12.14).

13. Hold wrist in one position and push wrist upwards, hold for 10 seconds and repeat × 10 × 2/day (Figure 12.15).
14. With weight in hand, rotate arm to left and right, repeat × 10 × 2 and do × 2/day (Figure 12.16).
15. Put toes onto small book, bend knee and stretch forward 10 × 15 second hold × 2/day (Figure 12.17).
16. With chin tucked in, rotate to right and hold × 5 seconds, repeat × 10 × 2/day (Figure 12.18).
17. With chin tucked in, rotate to left and hold × 5 seconds, repeat × 10 × 2/day (Figure 12.19).
18. Tuck chin in, repeat × 10 holding for 5 seconds (Figure 12.20).

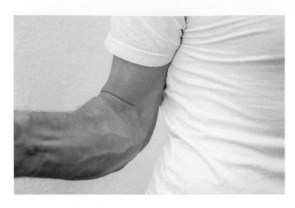

Figure 12.8 Shoulder extensor and lateral rotation strengthening.

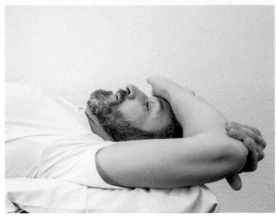

Figure 12.11 Shoulder capsule stretch.

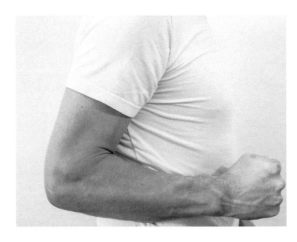

Figure 12.9 Shoulder extensor strengthening.

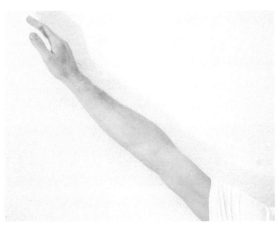

Figure 12.12 Wall walk for abduction.

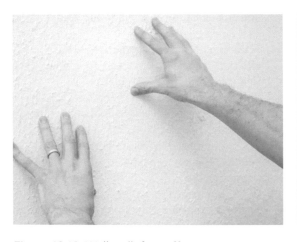

Figure 12.10 Wall walk for cuff tears.

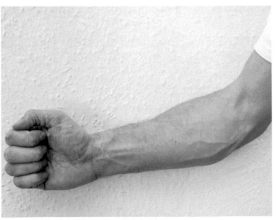

Figure 12.13 External rotation strengthening.

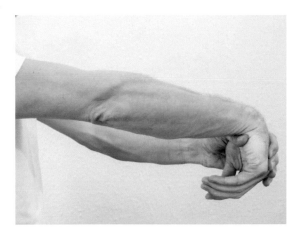

Figure 12.14 Extensor stretch lateral epicondylitis.

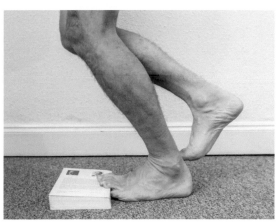

Figure 12.17 Toe flexor stretch.

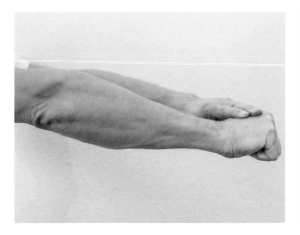

Figure 12.15 Isometric strengthening lateral epicondylitis.

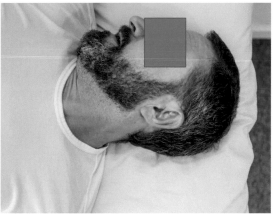

Figure 12.18 Chin tuck and rotation to right.

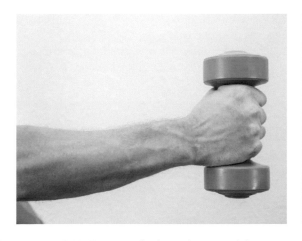

Figure 12.16 Rotation for lateral epicondylitis.

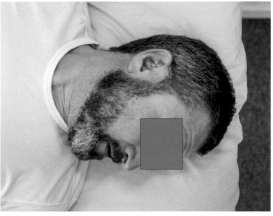

Figure 12.19 Chin tuck and rotation to left.

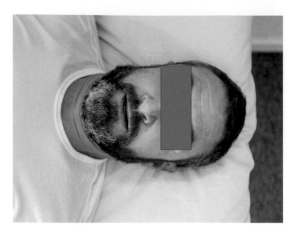

Figure 12.20 Chin tuck in lying.

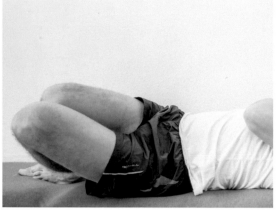

Figure 12.22 Lumbar spine – rotation to left.

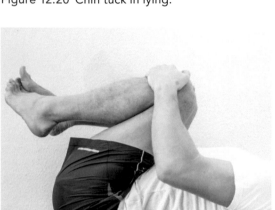

Figure 12.21 Lumbar spine – knees to chest.

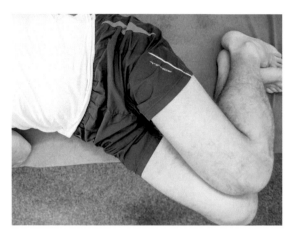

Figure 12.23 Lumbar spine – rotation to right.

19. Pull knees to chest × 10
    (hold 5 seconds) × 2/day (Figure 12.21).
20. Knee roll to left and right × 10 in each direction (hold at end for 2 seconds) × 2/day (Figure 12.22).
21. Knee roll to left and right × 10 in each direction (hold at end for 2 seconds) × 2/day (Figure 12.23).

## Resources

1. www.gpnotebook.co.uk
2. www.clinicalexam.com
3. www.patient.co.uk
4. *Clinical Examination* by Epstein O, Perkin G, Cookson J, de Bono D. 2003, London: Mosby Ltd

## SUMMARY

MSK disorders can be challenging to assess and treat. However, common conditions present in a familiar pattern. Accurate history taking and key examination findings will direct a clinician towards a diagnosis. Making a diagnosis, gaining trust by explaining the diagnosis combined with simple exercise prescription will invariably lead to improved patient satisfaction.

Patients who fall out of the 'familiar pattern' presentation may require further opinion and assessment.

5. *Macleod's Clinical Examination* by Douglas G, Nicol F, Robertson C. 2013, London: Churchill Livingston/Elsevier
6. *Clinical Examination: A Systemic Guide to Physical Diagnosis* by Talley N, O'Connor S. 2014, Chatswood, Australia: Churchill Livingstone/Elsevier

## References

1. Department of Health. *The Musculoskeletal Services Framework: A Joint Responsibility: Doing It Differently.* London: Department of Health, 2006, http://www.dh.gov.uk/prod consum dh/groups/dh digitalassets/@dh/@en/documents/digitalasset/dh 4138412.pdf

2. Arthritis Research UK National Primary Care Centre, Keele University. *Musculoskeletal Matters: What Do General Practitioners See.* Bulletin 1, Keele: Keele University, October 2009, http://www.keele.ac.uk/pchs/disseminatingourresearch/newslettersand resources/bulletins/bulletin1/

# 13

# Musculoskeletal disorders – the GP perspective

## TOM ROWLEY

## Introduction

Musculoskeletal (MSK) conditions are extremely common. Patients with these disorders fill our surgeries every day, with estimates suggesting they account for up to 30% of all general practitioner (GP) consultations. Whist rarely life threatening, they have a huge impact on the individual in terms of disability, well-being and fitness, as well as costs to society as a whole in respect of lost productivity, long-term sickness and National Health Service (NHS) resources.[1]

As a consequence, GP referrals to hospital outpatients for these conditions are invariably the highest across all specialties, resulting in long waiting times and pressures on an already overburdened system. And yet studies show that relatively few of these patients ever end up with a serious diagnosis or require surgical intervention.

The implication, therefore, is that a great many of our patients could be treated with less delay, more conveniently and more effectively within a primary care setting. All of which would result in much greater patient satisfaction and reduced costs to the NHS overall.

The barrier to this is that undergraduate training in MSK medicine remains woefully inadequate.[2] Most GP registrars, and even many experienced GPs, lack the clinical skills and confidence to diagnose and manage these patients effectively – an imbalance that the chapters in this book will hopefully go some way to address.

I have worked as a hospital practitioner in orthopaedics and as a GP with specialist interest in MSK for many years, but my main role and perspective is as a GP and a trainer. In this chapter, therefore, I aim to provide the generalist perspective, with an overview and a few key observations and principles. Some of these may already be familiar and self-evident to those of you who are more experienced, but I think they bear repeating.

## MSK conditions – the GP's essential role

When presenting to registrars or GP colleagues, the key message when seeing patients who present with MSK conditions, above all else, is – 'Do not miss serious disease'.

An accurate medical diagnosis has to come first, excluding cancer, infection, trauma, pathological fractures (not always acute) and inflammatory, vascular or serious neurological conditions. This is after all our prime role as doctors, but these conditions are often missed – careful history and examination in this respect are essential.

The most likely diagnosis in a 60-year-old woman presenting with an increasingly painful, stiff shoulder is adhesive capsulitis (frozen shoulder). However, a history of breast cancer diagnosed 9 months ago in this same patient changes everything.

Hopefully this book will allow you to diagnose MSK conditions with greater confidence, but if you do refer a patient with non-serious shoulder pain to one of your orthopaedic colleagues, and the eventual diagnosis turns out to be impingement rather than frozen shoulder, little harm is done – perhaps just a polite (hopefully!) letter to inform you. But refer our patient above with metastatic breast cancer to routine outpatients or physiotherapy, with long delays in diagnosis, and you can perhaps expect a very different set of letters.

## Red flags

You will have been aware of the system of red flags as applied to low-back pain before reading this book. Knowledge of these to screen for possible serious disease should be essential reading for all GPs.[3]

Although originally developed and intended for spinal pain, this approach can also be applied very effectively as a diagnostic 'grid' across the full range of MSK conditions that might present in your surgeries – the general principles are still relevant. Context and probability are important, and a common sense approach is needed. We don't have time in our busy surgeries to screen every patient extensively, and a fit 50-year-old man with typical symptoms of tennis elbow is likely to have just that, but awareness of the red flags should always be there on our radar, ready to apply whenever appropriate.

In areas of diagnostic uncertainty, especially where flags coexist, clarification of the duration and progression of symptoms can be useful and help discriminate. In an 80-year-old man with previous prostatic cancer, recent onset of progressively severe back pain is metastatic until proven otherwise, whereas a 2-year history of back pain in the same patient, unchanged and non-progressive over time, is less likely to be serious.

As doctors, we often talk about a 'sixth sense' that warns us when things aren't right. Of course, there is no such thing in reality – what we are actually responding to is based on experience, pattern recognition and a subconscious application of 'flags' like those above. Hoping that this sixth sense will always pop up to rescue us, however, is arbitrary and unreliable – far better to recognise and refine these same skills into a conscious, systematic approach. This gives us greater confidence in diagnosis and allows us to trust our judgement when we do need to act, even if all the tests have returned normal and we can't name what exactly is wrong.

## Clinical assessment – general principles

The chapters in this book have given descriptions in respect of specific orthopaedic and rheumatological conditions. My purpose in this section is to suggest some basic principles, with a general approach to MSK assessment you may find useful.

## History

- If you lack confidence in specific clinical examination skills, a careful history can help compensate and will very often identify the likely nature of the problem and a list of differential diagnoses. Done well, this alone should discriminate likely serious disease and rheumatological, vascular and neurological causes from mechanical MSK conditions. So often this step is rushed, with key points missed, making everything else so much harder.

- MSK conditions are primarily mechanical in nature. In your history, try to establish the underlying cause of the patients' symptoms, and what has led to them presenting now. Occupational and ergonomic factors, prolonged positions, repetitive use, training errors (excess loading/impact), technique (sports/musicians), footwear and intrinsic biomechanical factors (including weight gain) are all highly relevant. Specific enquiry here will not only help establish a diagnosis, but also allow a specific approach to treatment which will enable you to be far more effective in your management.

## Examination

Below are some key principles of MSK examination. These are based on work by Dr. James Cyriax, the 'father' of orthopaedic medicine. His book influenced me hugely when I read it many years ago, with the realisation that there was a simple diagnostic clinical approach that could be applied consistently. It is an easy read (pictures too!), and I recommend his first chapter on 'Principles of Diagnosis' as an introduction to you especially. A revision of regional local anatomy and the structures involved greatly assists.

## Approach to examination

- Fully expose the area to be examined: Above and below the area affected.
- Always compare and contrast both sides at all examination stages: This will help to identify minor differences that would otherwise be missed, e.g. subtle wasting/effusions.
- Inspection: All angles, consider biomechanics, compare and look carefully.
- Palpation: Targeted to anatomical structures and compare both sides for tenderness – localises specific structures and insertions involved.
- Active (patient) movements: E.g. painful arc, worthwhile but note that value is limited by pain, willingness and distress.
- Passive (examiner) movements: These are the essential discriminatory tests:
  - Must be tested to true end range and compared to normal side.
  - Any restriction, truly tested to end range, implies joint pathology (osteoarthritis [OA], rheumatoid arthritis [RA], frozen shoulder, loose body).
  - Hard end feel is typical of OA, soft can be meniscal or similar (or pain inhibition).
  - Each joint has a recognisable 'capsular' pattern: E.g. internal rotation most limited for hip, external rotation for shoulder.
  - End range passively stretches inert structures such as ligaments: E.g. anterior talofibular ligament (ATFL) in ankle strains.
  - Excessive range suggests joint laxity or rupture of passive restraints (e.g. anterior cruciate ligament [ACL] tests in the knee).
- Resisted movements test contractile structures: Muscles/tendons/insertions
  - Need to test in neutral mid-position (or joint/inert structures are stressed).
  - Direction of resistance that is painful/weak relates to mode of action of the affected structure so one can accurately localise and identify lesion.
  - Weak resisted tests may be due to pain inhibition (but patient can often overcome with instruction to allow valid test).
  - True weakness implies partial or full rupture of affected structure.
  - Marked weakness that is pain free can be full rupture, but think neurological also.
- Special tests: E.g. Hawkins impingement, McMurray, Lachman (just learn)
- Neurological: E.g. neural tension tests and straight leg raise (SLR) in sciatica
  - Always consider referred pain when local examination does not reveal a cause.
  - Pain tends to refer distally, e.g. knee pain from the hip, shoulder pain from the neck.
  - The opposite is not common: Trapezius pain is usually from the neck, thigh pain does not usually arise from the knee.
  - Nerve lesions: Clear boundaries and definition increases the more distal the lesion (e.g. carpal tunnel lesions vs. referred from neck).
- Vascular: Rarely needed but consider (e.g. foot pulses for claudication pattern).

The beauty of this system is that it is simple, consistent and can be applied effectively across the full range of MSK conditions you are likely to see. The principles involved provide a sound base on which to build the more detailed regional examination skills described in the previous chapters.

## Investigations

It is perhaps not surprising that in our busy GP surgeries, blood tests and x-rays are often requested after only the briefest of clinical assessments – a common shortcut, especially when we are running late and trying to catch up. However, MSK medicine is above all else a clinical specialty, and a good history and careful examination are far more important than any tests. Indeed, without clinical correlation, investigations can be highly misleading and often contribute to misdiagnosis and inappropriate referrals.

A history of early morning stiffness and small joint tenderness on examination is suggestive of inflammatory arthritis irrespective of blood tests. C-reactive protein (CRP) and autoantibodies can be normal, especially in seronegative arthritis. Rheumatoid factor and antinuclear antibody (ANA) are found in 5% of the population anyway, so checking them in a patient who clinically has OA only confuses. Serum urate can be both normal in patients with gout and raised in patients without it. I have seen classical polymyalgia with normal CRP and metastatic prostate cancer with normal prostate-specific antigen (PSA) (though alkaline phosphatase was raised).

Imaging is no exception – x-rays in early metastatic disease are frequently negative, ultrasound can show large rotator cuff tears in asymptomatic shoulders and magnetic resonance imaging (MRI) scans demonstrate significant disc pathology and protrusions in a high proportion of healthy asymptomatic volunteers.[4]

So the key message here is to avoid over-reliance on investigations – they should only be used in context and must be interpreted and correlated with careful clinical assessment.

## Management

So often in general practice, I see a standard response to the management of MSK conditions, that is 'rest and non-steroidal anti-inflammatory drugs (NSAIDs)'. Our patients must feel so underwhelmed leaving with just this advice – most of them will have waited and 'rested' before seeing us and many will have taken Ibuprofen over the counter anyway. We should do better than this.

Fortunately, there are again some key general principles and approaches to management that, with a little imagination, can be applied very effectively to most conditions you will see – a pick and mix list if you like.

## The MSK 'prescription'

- *Explanation:* Causes, biomechanical factors, training errors, ergonomics etc.
- *Advice:* Positive messages to maintain fitness and prevent deconditioning.
- The principle of *relative rest:* Initial protection and reduced stressing, followed by frequent, incremental, stepped activity guided by symptoms.

- *Specific rehabilitation:* Patient advice sheets for conditions (see Resources).
- *Formal physiotherapy referral* to supplement above.
- *Splints:* E.g. carpal tunnel and tennis elbow, but can also be useful to support weak/painful joints where other options are limited – e.g. knee and ankle braces.
- *Formal occupational therapy referral* to supplement above.
- *Footwear and insoles:* To offload, reduce impact and correct biomechanical factors such as pronation. Can help for all lower limbs, not just foot and ankle.
- *Formal podiatry/orthotic referral* to supplement above.
- *Medication:* Effective pain relief, prevents deconditioning and assists rehabilitation but far more effectively used as an adjunct to everything else, not in isolation.
  - Analgesia ladder, including NSAIDs, as per the National Institute for Health and Care Excellence (NICE) guidelines.
  - Topical NSAIDs: Especially for superficial joints.
  - Capsaicin cream: E.g. for knee OA but takes a few weeks for effectiveness.
  - Neuropathic medications: E.g. tricyclics, gabapentin and pregablin. Can be very effective but dose titration and counsel patients can take weeks to work.
- *Steroid injections:* See below.
- *Further investigation/imaging:* Mentioned here because often what many patients want is a definitive diagnosis rather than surgical intervention.
- *Orthopaedic referral*
  - Complex diagnoses, further investigation, expert opinion and management.
  - Surgical intervention: But discuss! Many patients attending outpatients don't actually want an operation when all the risks are fully explained.
- *Rheumatology referral:* Should be early if inflammatory disease is suspected.

It is simple to apply these general principles as a checklist, adapting and using it to build individualised and specific treatment plans for the patients you see – far more impressive than just rest and NSAIDs.

# Steroid injections in primary care

Injections are commonly used in primary care and can undoubtedly be very effective. With appropriate training and case selection, they are of low risk. Infection is what everyone worries about, but is far less common than many think – estimates put this at around 1:30,000 for those performed in general practice. The risk I worry about is tendon rupture. Flushing and post-injection flare are common, however, and the patient does need to be counselled about these.

The safety record of injections should certainly be considered in respect of NSAIDs which we as GPs prescribe all the time – quick and easy to dispense, but with a much higher risk profile, including serious complications, hospital admission and even death.

Injection skills can be readily learned. Many orthopaedic departments run regular training sessions, and there are excellent practical guides that can be used for reference.

There are a number of important considerations that are worth emphasising which are as follows:

- Good training is essential: Both procedural skills and assessment of risks/contraindications.
- Injections should be only considered as an adjunct to other treatments: They relieve pain and inflammation, but don't address the underlying causes and pathology.
- Ignore this and you will find short-term relief, but your patients will come back.[5]
- Acquiring confidence to put a needle in is the easy part. The skill is the accurate diagnosis and appropriate case selection to ensure you identify those patients who are safe, appropriate and likely to respond.
- Stay within your comfort zone: Choose a few 'quick wins' and stick with them.

Choice of injection procedures – this would be how I would summarise the most common GP injections.

- *Technically easy and usually good response*
  - Shoulder subacromial injection
  - Trochanteric bursitis (less so if significant OA back/hip associated)

- *Technically easy and can be useful but often short-term benefit only*
  - Tennis/golfer's elbow
  - OA knee
- *Less easy technically but can be very effective*
  - Shoulder AC joint
  - Carpometacarpal (CMC) (thumb) and metatarsophalangeal (MTP) (hallux) joints
  - De Quervain's and trigger finger
- *Less easy technically and variable outcome but worthwhile*
  - Frozen shoulder (treatment of choice in early inflammatory stage)
  - Carpal tunnel syndrome (effective in mild cases if other factors addressed)
- *Ones to avoid*
  - High weight/load bearing tendons, e.g. Achilles/patellar/tibialis posterior
  - Younger patients: Establish clear diagnosis, injections often inappropriate

# Physiotherapy

The key message here is that not all physiotherapy is the same. Levels of specific training, experience, areas of interest and specialisation vary widely. Not infrequently, treatment failure can be simply because your patient has not seen the most appropriate practitioner. Impingement syndrome in a young patient, for example, is often due to complex instability and needs specific expertise to address. Always enquire about the treatment received – is it specific and appropriate to the patient's condition? Ultrasound and other esoteric 'black box' electrical treatments are highly suspect – discount these and re-refer. Most large NHS departments should triage referrals effectively in this respect, but this is not always the case. Small local departments may be more limited in their resources, and independent private practitioners vary widely.

As GPs, the standard perception and use of physiotherapy are resources we refer our patients to for treatment. This is undoubtedly a key core service, but I believe we are missing an opportunity in primary care, by not finding imaginative ways to extend their role further. The use of nurse practitioners in GP surgeries is well established (we use them too), so why not more extended scope physiotherapists? This makes perfect sense considering the high proportion of MSK-related conditions which otherwise use up limited doctor appointments, especially with the current difficulties in GP recruitment.

Our practice employs two of these experienced extended scope practitioners (ESPs) in place of a salaried GP. Their role is not to provide standard physiotherapy treatment, but to triage, diagnose and manage patients who would otherwise book with a GP. They perform most of the injections within the practice, request further imaging when needed and refer on to secondary care when appropriate. They have 10-minute appointments, need very little back-up and are actually far better at this than most GPs are – doctors in our practice refer to them for second opinions. Although not 'medical', they are highly experienced at identifying atypical MSK presentations also, so very effective at screening out potentially serious disease – a crucial role when working in this capacity.

There is potential for greater use of this in primary care – our service is efficient, well-liked by patients and economically viable (when the alternative is additional salaried doctor sessions). Careful selection is essential, however, since only very experienced practitioners can work independently and safely in this role – they are a relatively scarce resource also at this level.

---

## SUMMARY POINTS

MSK presentations are common in our everyday practice, and yet these patients are often served poorly by GPs lacking expertise and adequate training. In this chapter, I have tried to show how a few general principles and a consistent approach can be applied effectively to many of the conditions you will see. Most patients will not benefit greatly from the prescription pad or need referral to secondary care, and only a few will want surgical intervention. A confident diagnosis, specific advice and explanation, positive messages and an individualised approach to rehabilitation and management is what our patients really want. This is where the 'Art' of MSK medicine is to be found in general practice – apply this and hopefully you will find it makes a big difference to how your patients leave the room at the end of your consultation.

---

## Resources

Two essential skills as GPs we attain with experience – learning to recognise when we don't know something and knowing where to look to find out. Our current orthopaedic and rheumatology consultant colleagues are most approachable, but we can't ring them or their busy registrars up too often.

Below I have given a list of resources you may find helpful. I must stress that this is not intended to be a definitive list – there will be omissions. Below I have given a list of resources you may find helpful. I must stress that this is not intended to be a definitive list - there will be omissions. So please consider this more as a personal selection that you might find useful as a starting point to then build on and create your own.

- *General texts and reference:*
  - *Cyriax's Illustrated Manual of Orthopaedic Medicine*, by James H. Cyriax
  - *Brukner & Khan's Clinical Sports Medicine*, 4th edition by Peter Brukner and Karim Khan (my 'must have' clinical text for MSK/sports)
  - *Colour Atlas of Human Anatomy: Vol. 1: Locomotor System* by Werner Platzer, 2014 (much more practical than Gray's)
  - *Apley and Solomon's Concise System of Orthopaedics and Trauma*, 4th edition by Louis Solomon, David Warwick and Selvadurai Nayagam, 2014
  - *Oxford Textbook of Musculoskeletal Medicine* by Michael Hutson and Richard Ellis, 2015
  - *Musculoskeletal Disorders in Primary Care (RCGP Curriculum for General Practice),* April 2012 by Louise Warburton (Editor)
- *Clinical assessment/skills:*
  - http://elearning.rcgp.org.uk/course/info.php?id=118&nopopup=1
  - http://www.arthritisresearchuk.org/health-professionals-and-students/student-handbook.aspx
- *Organisations and societies:*
  - Primary Care Rheumatology Society, https://www.pcrsociety.org/
  - ARUK, http://www.arthritisresearchuk.org/
  - British Rheumatology Society, https://www.pcrsociety.org/
  - BIMM, http://www.bimm.org.uk/
  - BASEM, http://www.basem.co.uk/

- *MSK/sports and rheumatology further training:*
  - PCR/Bradford Diploma in Musculoskeletal Medicine with Rheumatology, http://www.educationprogrammes.bradford.nhs.uk/Pages/MSK.aspx
  - MSc/PGDip Diploma in Musculoskeletal Medicine, http://www.lboro.ac.uk/study/postgraduate/programmes/departments/ssehs/musculoskeletal-medicine/
  - National Association of Sports and Exercise Medicine MSc/PGDip Diploma, http://www.ncsem-em.org.uk/education/msk-medicine/
  - BASEM MSc/Diploma Examination in Sport and Exercise Medicine/Science, http://www.basem.co.uk/education/mscdiploma-examination-in-sport-and-exercise-medicine.html
- *Joint injections:*
  - *Injection Techniques in Musculoskeletal Medicine: A Practical Manual for Clinicians in Primary and Secondary Care*, 4th edition by Stephanie Saunders and Steve Longworth (great practical manual clinical features, anatomy and injection technique with diagrams)
- *Rehabilitation advice and resources:*
  - http://www.arthritisresearchuk.org/health-professionals-and-students/information-for-your-patients/exercise-sheets-and-videos.aspx
  - http://www.physiotools.com/# excellent detailed resource but subscription
  - *Sports Medicine Patient Advisor Paperback March 2010* by Pierre Rouzier (rehabilitation advice sheets for conditions to be copied out for patients)
  - http://www.elht.nhs.uk/departments-wards-and-services/new_page_5.htm

(an example of some of the resources from local services that can be found – this one from Lancashire)
- http://www.keele.ac.uk/sbst/ (STarT Back is a stratified care approach and simple tool for back pain to match patients to most appropriate management.)

## References

1. Department of Health. *The Musculoskeletal Services Framework. A joint responsibility: Doing it differently.* London: Department of Health, 12 July 2006, http://webarchive.nationalarchives.gov.uk/20130107105354/http:/www.dh.gov.uk/prod_consum_dh/groups/dh_digitalassets/@dh/@en/documents/digitalasset/dh_4.
2. Al-Nammari SS, Pengas I, Asopa V, Jawad A Rafferty M, Ramachandran M. The inadequacy of musculoskeletal knowledge in graduating medical students in the United Kingdom. *J Bone Joint Surg Am.* 2015 Apr 1;97(7):e36. doi: 10.2106/JBJS.N.00488
3. Samanta J, Kendall J, Samanta A. 10-minute consultation: Chronic low back pain. *BMJ.* 2003;326:535. http://www.bmj.com/content/326/7388/535
4. Jensen MC, Brant-Zawadzki MN, Obuchowski N, Modic MT, Malkasian D, Ross JS. Magnetic resonance imaging of the lumbar spine in people without back pain. *N Engl J Med.* 1994;331:69–73.
5. Coombes BK, Bisset L, Brooks P, Khan A, Vicenzino B. Effect of corticosteroid injection, physiotherapy, or both on clinical outcomes in patients with unilateral lateral epicondylalgia: A randomized controlled trial. *JAMA.* 2013;309(5):461–469.

# Index